RHIT
Exam

SECRETS

Study Guide
Your Key to Exam Success

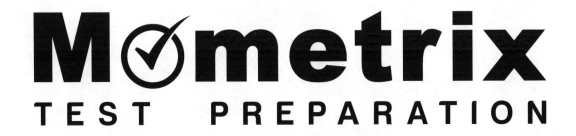

DEAR FUTURE EXAM SUCCESS STORY

First of all, **THANK YOU** for purchasing Mometrix study materials!

Second, congratulations! You are one of the few determined test-takers who are committed to doing whatever it takes to excel on your exam. **You have come to the right place.** We developed these study materials with one goal in mind: to deliver you the information you need in a format that's concise and easy to use.

In addition to optimizing your guide for the content of the test, we've outlined our recommended steps for breaking down the preparation process into small, attainable goals so you can make sure you stay on track.

We've also analyzed the entire test-taking process, identifying the most common pitfalls and showing how you can overcome them and be ready for any curveball the test throws you.

Standardized testing is one of the biggest obstacles on your road to success, which only increases the importance of doing well in the high-pressure, high-stakes environment of test day. Your results on this test could have a significant impact on your future, and this guide provides the information and practical advice to help you achieve your full potential on test day.

Your success is our success

We would love to hear from you! If you would like to share the story of your exam success or if you have any questions or comments in regard to our products, please contact us at **800-673-8175** or **support@mometrix.com**.

Thanks again for your business and we wish you continued success!

Sincerely,
The Mometrix Test Preparation Team

Need more help? Check out our flashcards at:
http://MometrixFlashcards.com/AHIMA

TABLE OF CONTENTS

INTRODUCTION _____ 1

SECRET KEY #1 – PLAN BIG, STUDY SMALL _____ 2

SECRET KEY #2 – MAKE YOUR STUDYING COUNT _____ 4

SECRET KEY #3 – PRACTICE THE RIGHT WAY _____ 6

SECRET KEY #4 – PACE YOURSELF _____ 8

SECRET KEY #5 – HAVE A PLAN FOR GUESSING _____ 9

TEST-TAKING STRATEGIES _____ 12

DATA CONTENT, STRUCTURE, AND INFORMATION GOVERNANCE _____ 17

ACCESS, DISCLOSURE, PRIVACY, AND SECURITY _____ 37

DATA ANALYTICS AND USE _____ 48

REVENUE CYCLE MANAGEMENT _____ 63

COMPLIANCE _____ 86

LEADERSHIP _____ 96

RHIT PRACTICE TEST _____ 102

ANSWER KEY AND EXPLANATIONS _____ 111

HOW TO OVERCOME TEST ANXIETY _____ 122
    CAUSES OF TEST ANXIETY _____ 122
    ELEMENTS OF TEST ANXIETY _____ 123
    EFFECTS OF TEST ANXIETY _____ 123
    PHYSICAL STEPS FOR BEATING TEST ANXIETY _____ 124
    MENTAL STEPS FOR BEATING TEST ANXIETY _____ 125
    STUDY STRATEGY _____ 126
    TEST TIPS _____ 128
    IMPORTANT QUALIFICATION _____ 129

THANK YOU _____ 130

ADDITIONAL BONUS MATERIAL _____ 131

Introduction

Thank you for purchasing this resource! You have made the choice to prepare yourself for a test that could have a huge impact on your future, and this guide is designed to help you be fully ready for test day. Obviously, it's important to have a solid understanding of the test material, but you also need to be prepared for the unique environment and stressors of the test, so that you can perform to the best of your abilities.

For this purpose, the first section that appears in this guide is the **Secret Keys**. We've devoted countless hours to meticulously researching what works and what doesn't, and we've boiled down our findings to the five most impactful steps you can take to improve your performance on the test. We start at the beginning with study planning and move through the preparation process, all the way to the testing strategies that will help you get the most out of what you know when you're finally sitting in front of the test.

We recommend that you start preparing for your test as far in advance as possible. However, if you've bought this guide as a last-minute study resource and only have a few days before your test, we recommend that you skip over the first two Secret Keys since they address a long-term study plan.

If you struggle with **test anxiety**, we strongly encourage you to check out our recommendations for how you can overcome it. Test anxiety is a formidable foe, but it can be beaten, and we want to make sure you have the tools you need to defeat it.

Secret Key #1 – Plan Big, Study Small

There's a lot riding on your performance. If you want to ace this test, you're going to need to keep your skills sharp and the material fresh in your mind. You need a plan that lets you review everything you need to know while still fitting in your schedule. We'll break this strategy down into three categories.

Information Organization

Start with the information you already have: the official test outline. From this, you can make a complete list of all the concepts you need to cover before the test. Organize these concepts into groups that can be studied together, and create a list of any related vocabulary you need to learn so you can brush up on any difficult terms. You'll want to keep this vocabulary list handy once you actually start studying since you may need to add to it along the way.

Time Management

Once you have your set of study concepts, decide how to spread them out over the time you have left before the test. Break your study plan into small, clear goals so you have a manageable task for each day and know exactly what you're doing. Then just focus on one small step at a time. When you manage your time this way, you don't need to spend hours at a time studying. Studying a small block of content for a short period each day helps you retain information better and avoid stressing over how much you have left to do. You can relax knowing that you have a plan to cover everything in time. In order for this strategy to be effective though, you have to start studying early and stick to your schedule. Avoid the exhaustion and futility that comes from last-minute cramming!

Study Environment

The environment you study in has a big impact on your learning. Studying in a coffee shop, while probably more enjoyable, is not likely to be as fruitful as studying in a quiet room. It's important to keep distractions to a minimum. You're only planning to study for a short block of time, so make the most of it. Don't pause to check your phone or get up to find a snack. It's also important to **avoid multitasking**. Research has consistently shown that multitasking will make your studying dramatically less effective. Your study area should also be comfortable and well-lit so you don't have the distraction of straining your eyes or sitting on an uncomfortable chair.

The time of day you study is also important. You want to be rested and alert. Don't wait until just before bedtime. Study when you'll be most likely to comprehend and remember. Even better, if you know what time of day your test will be, set that time aside for study. That way your brain will be used to working on that subject at that specific time and you'll have a better chance of recalling information.

Finally, it can be helpful to team up with others who are studying for the same test. Your actual studying should be done in as isolated an environment as possible, but the work of organizing the information and setting up the study plan can be divided up. In between study sessions, you can discuss with your teammates the concepts that you're all studying and quiz each other on the details. Just be sure that your teammates are as serious about the test as you are. If you find that your study time is being replaced with social time, you might need to find a new team.

Secret Key #2 – Make Your Studying Count

You're devoting a lot of time and effort to preparing for this test, so you want to be absolutely certain it will pay off. This means doing more than just reading the content and hoping you can remember it on test day. It's important to make every minute of study count. There are two main areas you can focus on to make your studying count:

Retention

It doesn't matter how much time you study if you can't remember the material. You need to make sure you are retaining the concepts. To check your retention of the information you're learning, try recalling it at later times with minimal prompting. Try carrying around flashcards and glance at one or two from time to time or ask a friend who's also studying for the test to quiz you.

To enhance your retention, look for ways to put the information into practice so that you can apply it rather than simply recalling it. If you're using the information in practical ways, it will be much easier to remember. Similarly, it helps to solidify a concept in your mind if you're not only reading it to yourself but also explaining it to someone else. Ask a friend to let you teach them about a concept you're a little shaky on (or speak aloud to an imaginary audience if necessary). As you try to summarize, define, give examples, and answer your friend's questions, you'll understand the concepts better and they will stay with you longer. Finally, step back for a big picture view and ask yourself how each piece of information fits with the whole subject. When you link the different concepts together and see them working together as a whole, it's easier to remember the individual components.

Finally, practice showing your work on any multi-step problems, even if you're just studying. Writing out each step you take to solve a problem will help solidify the process in your mind, and you'll be more likely to remember it during the test.

Modality

Modality simply refers to the means or method by which you study. Choosing a study modality that fits your own individual learning style is crucial. No two people learn best in exactly the same way, so it's important to know your strengths and use them to your advantage.

For example, if you learn best by visualization, focus on visualizing a concept in your mind and draw an image or a diagram. Try color-coding your notes, illustrating them, or creating symbols that will trigger your mind to recall a learned concept. If you learn best by hearing or discussing information, find a study partner who learns the same way or read aloud to yourself. Think about how to put the information in

4

your own words. Imagine that you are giving a lecture on the topic and record yourself so you can listen to it later.

For any learning style, flashcards can be helpful. Organize the information so you can take advantage of spare moments to review. Underline key words or phrases. Use different colors for different categories. Mnemonic devices (such as creating a short list in which every item starts with the same letter) can also help with retention. Find what works best for you and use it to store the information in your mind most effectively and easily.

Secret Key #3 – Practice the Right Way

Your success on test day depends not only on how many hours you put into preparing, but also on whether you prepared the right way. It's good to check along the way to see if your studying is paying off. One of the most effective ways to do this is by taking practice tests to evaluate your progress. Practice tests are useful because they show exactly where you need to improve. Every time you take a practice test, pay special attention to these three groups of questions:

- The questions you got wrong
- The questions you had to guess on, even if you guessed right
- The questions you found difficult or slow to work through

This will show you exactly what your weak areas are, and where you need to devote more study time. Ask yourself why each of these questions gave you trouble. Was it because you didn't understand the material? Was it because you didn't remember the vocabulary? Do you need more repetitions on this type of question to build speed and confidence? Dig into those questions and figure out how you can strengthen your weak areas as you go back to review the material.

Additionally, many practice tests have a section explaining the answer choices. It can be tempting to read the explanation and think that you now have a good understanding of the concept. However, an explanation likely only covers part of the question's broader context. Even if the explanation makes sense, **go back and investigate** every concept related to the question until you're positive you have a thorough understanding.

As you go along, keep in mind that the practice test is just that: practice. Memorizing these questions and answers will not be very helpful on the actual test because it is unlikely to have any of the same exact questions. If you only know the right answers to the sample questions, you won't be prepared for the real thing. **Study the concepts** until you understand them fully, and then you'll be able to answer any question that shows up on the test.

It's important to wait on the practice tests until you're ready. If you take a test on your first day of study, you may be overwhelmed by the amount of material covered and how much you need to learn. Work up to it gradually.

On test day, you'll need to be prepared for answering questions, managing your time, and using the test-taking strategies you've learned. It's a lot to balance, like a mental marathon that will have a big impact on your future. Like training for a marathon, you'll need to start slowly and work your way up. When test day arrives, you'll be ready.

Start with the strategies you've read in the first two Secret Keys—plan your course and study in the way that works best for you. If you have time, consider using multiple study resources to get different approaches to the same concepts. It can be helpful to see difficult concepts from more than one angle. Then find a good source for practice tests. Many times, the test website will suggest potential study resources or provide sample tests.

Practice Test Strategy

If you're able to find at least three practice tests, we recommend this strategy:

1. Take the first test with no time constraints and with your notes and study guide handy. Take your time and focus on applying the strategies you've learned.
2. Take the second practice test open-book as well, but set a timer and practice pacing yourself to finish in time.
3. Take any other practice tests as if it were test day. Set a timer and put away your study materials. Sit at a table or desk in a quiet room, imagine yourself at the testing center, and answer questions as quickly and accurately as possible.
4. Keep repeating step 3 on a regular basis until you run out of practice tests or it's time for the actual test. Your mind will be ready for the schedule and stress of test day, and you'll be able to focus on recalling the material you've learned.

Secret Key #4 – Pace Yourself

Once you're fully prepared for the material on the test, your biggest challenge on test day will be managing your time. Just knowing that the clock is ticking can make you panic even if you have plenty of time left. Work on pacing yourself so you can build confidence against the time constraints of the exam. Pacing is a difficult skill to master, especially in a high-pressure environment, so **practice is vital**.

Set time expectations for your pace based on how much time is available. For example, if a section has 60 questions and the time limit is 30 minutes, you know you have to average 30 seconds or less per question in order to answer them all. Although 30 seconds is the hard limit, set 25 seconds per question as your goal, so you reserve extra time to spend on harder questions. When you budget extra time for the harder questions, you no longer have any reason to stress when those questions take longer to answer.

Don't let this time expectation distract you from working through the test at a calm, steady pace, but keep it in mind so you don't spend too much time on any one question. Recognize that taking extra time on one question you don't understand may keep you from answering two that you do understand later in the test. If your time limit for a question is up and you're still not sure of the answer, mark it and move on, and come back to it later if the time and the test format allow. If the testing format doesn't allow you to return to earlier questions, just make an educated guess; then put it out of your mind and move on.

On the easier questions, be careful not to rush. It may seem wise to hurry through them so you have more time for the challenging ones, but it's not worth missing one if you know the concept and just didn't take the time to read the question fully. Work efficiently but make sure you understand the question and have looked at all of the answer choices, since more than one may seem right at first.

Even if you're paying attention to the time, you may find yourself a little behind at some point. You should speed up to get back on track, but do so wisely. Don't panic; just take a few seconds less on each question until you're caught up. Don't guess without thinking, but do look through the answer choices and eliminate any you know are wrong. If you can get down to two choices, it is often worthwhile to guess from those. Once you've chosen an answer, move on and don't dwell on any that you skipped or had to hurry through. If a question was taking too long, chances are it was one of the harder ones, so you weren't as likely to get it right anyway.

On the other hand, if you find yourself getting ahead of schedule, it may be beneficial to slow down a little. The more quickly you work, the more likely you are to make a careless mistake that will affect your score. You've budgeted time for each question, so don't be afraid to spend that time. Practice an efficient but careful pace to get the most out of the time you have.

8

Secret Key #5 – Have a Plan for Guessing

When you're taking the test, you may find yourself stuck on a question. Some of the answer choices seem better than others, but you don't see the one answer choice that is obviously correct. What do you do?

The scenario described above is very common, yet most test takers have not effectively prepared for it. Developing and practicing a plan for guessing may be one of the single most effective uses of your time as you get ready for the exam.

In developing your plan for guessing, there are three questions to address:

- When should you start the guessing process?
- How should you narrow down the choices?
- Which answer should you choose?

When to Start the Guessing Process

Unless your plan for guessing is to select C every time (which, despite its merits, is not what we recommend), you need to leave yourself enough time to apply your answer elimination strategies. Since you have a limited amount of time for each question, that means that if you're going to give yourself the best shot at guessing correctly, you have to decide quickly whether or not you will guess.

Of course, the best-case scenario is that you don't have to guess at all, so first, see if you can answer the question based on your knowledge of the subject and basic reasoning skills. Focus on the key words in the question and try to jog your memory of related topics. Give yourself a chance to bring the knowledge to mind, but once you realize that you don't have (or you can't access) the knowledge you need to answer the question, it's time to start the guessing process.

It's almost always better to start the guessing process too early than too late. It only takes a few seconds to remember something and answer the question from knowledge. Carefully eliminating wrong answer choices takes longer. Plus, going through the process of eliminating answer choices can actually help jog your memory.

Summary: Start the guessing process as soon as you decide that you can't answer the question based on your knowledge.

9

How to Narrow Down the Choices

The next chapter in this book (**Test-Taking Strategies**) includes a wide range of strategies for how to approach questions and how to look for answer choices to eliminate. You will definitely want to read those carefully, practice them, and figure out which ones work best for you. Here though, we're going to address a mindset rather than a particular strategy.

Your chances of guessing an answer correctly depend on how many options you are choosing from.

How many choices you have	How likely you are to guess correctly
5	20%
4	25%
3	33%
2	50%
1	100%

You can see from this chart just how valuable it is to be able to eliminate incorrect answers and make an educated guess, but there are two things that many test takers do that cause them to miss out on the benefits of guessing:

- Accidentally eliminating the correct answer
- Selecting an answer based on an impression

We'll look at the first one here, and the second one in the next section.

To avoid accidentally eliminating the correct answer, we recommend a thought exercise called **the $5 challenge**. In this challenge, you only eliminate an answer choice from contention if you are willing to bet $5 on it being wrong. Why $5? Five dollars is a small but not insignificant amount of money. It's an amount you could afford to lose but wouldn't want to throw away. And while losing $5 once might not hurt too much, doing it twenty times will set you back $100. In the same way, each small decision you make—eliminating a choice here, guessing on a question there—won't by itself impact your score very much, but when you put them all together, they can make a big difference. By holding each answer choice elimination decision to a higher standard, you can reduce the risk of accidentally eliminating the correct answer.

The $5 challenge can also be applied in a positive sense: If you are willing to bet $5 that an answer choice *is* correct, go ahead and mark it as correct.

Summary: Only eliminate an answer choice if you are willing to bet $5 that it is wrong.

Which Answer to Choose

You're taking the test. You've run into a hard question and decided you'll have to guess. You've eliminated all the answer choices you're willing to bet $5 on. Now you have to pick an answer. Why do we even need to talk about this? Why can't you just pick whichever one you feel like when the time comes?

The answer to these questions is that if you don't come into the test with a plan, you'll rely on your impression to select an answer choice, and if you do that, you risk falling into a trap. The test writers know that everyone who takes their test will be guessing on some of the questions, so they intentionally write wrong answer choices to seem plausible. You still have to pick an answer though, and if the wrong answer choices are designed to look right, how can you ever be sure that you're not falling for their trap? The best solution we've found to this dilemma is to take the decision out of your hands entirely. Here is the process we recommend:

Once you've eliminated any choices that you are confident (willing to bet $5) are wrong, select the first remaining choice as your answer.

Whether you choose to select the first remaining choice, the second, or the last, the important thing is that you use some preselected standard. Using this approach guarantees that you will not be enticed into selecting an answer choice that looks right, because you are not basing your decision on how the answer choices look.

This is not meant to make you question your knowledge. Instead, it is to help you recognize the difference between your knowledge and your impressions. There's a huge difference between thinking an answer is right because of what you know, and thinking an answer is right because it looks or sounds like it should be right.

Summary: To ensure that your selection is appropriately random, make a predetermined selection from among all answer choices you have not eliminated.

Test-Taking Strategies

This section contains a list of test-taking strategies that you may find helpful as you work through the test. By taking what you know and applying logical thought, you can maximize your chances of answering any question correctly!

It is very important to realize that every question is different and every person is different: no single strategy will work on every question, and no single strategy will work for every person. That's why we've included all of them here, so you can try them out and determine which ones work best for different types of questions and which ones work best for you.

Question Strategies

READ CAREFULLY

Read the question and answer choices carefully. Don't miss the question because you misread the terms. You have plenty of time to read each question thoroughly and make sure you understand what is being asked. Yet a happy medium must be attained, so don't waste too much time. You must read carefully, but efficiently.

CONTEXTUAL CLUES

Look for contextual clues. If the question includes a word you are not familiar with, look at the immediate context for some indication of what the word might mean. Contextual clues can often give you all the information you need to decipher the meaning of an unfamiliar word. Even if you can't determine the meaning, you may be able to narrow down the possibilities enough to make a solid guess at the answer to the question.

PREFIXES

If you're having trouble with a word in the question or answer choices, try dissecting it. Take advantage of every clue that the word might include. Prefixes and suffixes can be a huge help. Usually they allow you to determine a basic meaning. Pre- means before, post- means after, pro - is positive, de- is negative. From prefixes and suffixes, you can get an idea of the general meaning of the word and try to put it into context.

HEDGE WORDS

Watch out for critical hedge words, such as *likely, may, can, sometimes, often, almost, mostly, usually, generally, rarely*, and *sometimes*. Question writers insert these hedge phrases to cover every possibility. Often an answer choice will be wrong simply because it leaves no room for exception. Be on guard for answer choices that have definitive words such as *exactly* and *always*.

SWITCHBACK WORDS

Stay alert for *switchbacks*. These are the words and phrases frequently used to alert you to shifts in thought. The most common switchback words are *but, although*, and *however*. Others include *nevertheless, on the other hand, even though, while, in spite of, despite, regardless of*. Switchback words are important to catch because they can change the direction of the question or an answer choice.

FACE VALUE

When in doubt, use common sense. Accept the situation in the problem at face value. Don't read too much into it. These problems will not require you to make wild assumptions. If you have to go beyond creativity and warp time or space in order to have an answer choice fit the question, then you should move on and consider the other answer choices. These are normal problems rooted in reality. The applicable relationship or explanation may not be readily apparent, but it is there for you to figure out. Use your common sense to interpret anything that isn't clear.

Answer Choice Strategies

ANSWER SELECTION

The most thorough way to pick an answer choice is to identify and eliminate wrong answers until only one is left, then confirm it is the correct answer. Sometimes an answer choice may immediately seem right, but be careful. The test writers will usually put more than one reasonable answer choice on each question, so take a second to read all of them and make sure that the other choices are not equally obvious. As long as you have time left, it is better to read every answer choice than to pick the first one that looks right without checking the others.

ANSWER CHOICE FAMILIES

An answer choice family consists of two (in rare cases, three) answer choices that are very similar in construction and cannot all be true at the same time. If you see two answer choices that are direct opposites or parallels, one of them is usually the correct answer. For instance, if one answer choice says that quantity x increases and another either says that quantity x decreases (opposite) or says that quantity y increases (parallel), then those answer choices would fall into the same family. An answer choice that doesn't match the construction of the answer choice family is more likely to be incorrect. Most questions will not have answer choice families, but when they do appear, you should be prepared to recognize them.

ELIMINATE ANSWERS

Eliminate answer choices as soon as you realize they are wrong, but make sure you consider all possibilities. If you are eliminating answer choices and realize that the last one you are left with is also wrong, don't panic. Start over and consider each choice again. There may be something you missed the first time that you will realize on the second pass.

AVOID FACT TRAPS

Don't be distracted by an answer choice that is factually true but doesn't answer the question. You are looking for the choice that answers the question. Stay focused on what the question is asking for so you don't accidentally pick an answer that is true but incorrect. Always go back to the question and make sure the answer choice you've selected actually answers the question and is not merely a true statement.

EXTREME STATEMENTS

In general, you should avoid answers that put forth extreme actions as standard practice or proclaim controversial ideas as established fact. An answer choice that states the "process should be used in certain situations, if..." is much more likely to be correct than one that states the "process should be discontinued completely." The first is a calm rational statement and doesn't even make a definitive, uncompromising stance, using a hedge word *if* to provide wiggle room, whereas the second choice is a radical idea and far more extreme.

BENCHMARK

As you read through the answer choices and you come across one that seems to answer the question well, mentally select that answer choice. This is not your final answer, but it's the one that will help you evaluate the other answer choices. The one that you selected is your benchmark or standard for judging each of the other answer choices. Every other answer choice must be compared to your benchmark. That choice is correct until proven otherwise by another answer choice beating it. If you find a better answer, then that one becomes your new benchmark. Once you've decided that no other choice answers the question as well as your benchmark, you have your final answer.

PREDICT THE ANSWER

Before you even start looking at the answer choices, it is often best to try to predict the answer. When you come up with the answer on your own, it is easier to avoid distractions and traps because you will know exactly what to look for. The right answer choice is unlikely to be word-for-word what you came up with, but it should be a close match. Even if you are confident that you have the right answer, you should still take the time to read each option before moving on.

General Strategies

TOUGH QUESTIONS

If you are stumped on a problem or it appears too hard or too difficult, don't waste time. Move on! Remember though, if you can quickly check for obviously incorrect answer choices, your chances of guessing correctly are greatly improved. Before you completely give up, at least try to knock out a couple of possible answers. Eliminate what you can and then guess at the remaining answer choices before moving on.

14

CHECK YOUR WORK

Since you will probably not know every term listed and the answer to every question, it is important that you get credit for the ones that you do know. Don't miss any questions through careless mistakes. If at all possible, try to take a second to look back over your answer selection and make sure you've selected the correct answer choice and haven't made a costly careless mistake (such as marking an answer choice that you didn't mean to mark). This quick double check should more than pay for itself in caught mistakes for the time it costs.

PACE YOURSELF

It's easy to be overwhelmed when you're looking at a page full of questions; your mind is confused and full of random thoughts, and the clock is ticking down faster than you would like. Calm down and maintain the pace that you have set for yourself. Especially as you get down to the last few minutes of the test, don't let the small numbers on the clock make you panic. As long as you are on track by monitoring your pace, you are guaranteed to have time for each question.

DON'T RUSH

It is very easy to make errors when you are in a hurry. Maintaining a fast pace in answering questions is pointless if it makes you miss questions that you would have gotten right otherwise. Test writers like to include distracting information and wrong answers that seem right. Taking a little extra time to avoid careless mistakes can make all the difference in your test score. Find a pace that allows you to be confident in the answers that you select.

KEEP MOVING

Panicking will not help you pass the test, so do your best to stay calm and keep moving. Taking deep breaths and going through the answer elimination steps you practiced can help to break through a stress barrier and keep your pace.

Final Notes

The combination of a solid foundation of content knowledge and the confidence that comes from practicing your plan for applying that knowledge is the key to maximizing your performance on test day. As your foundation of content knowledge is built up and strengthened, you'll find that the strategies included in this chapter become more and more effective in helping you quickly sift through the distractions and traps of the test to isolate the correct answer.

Now it's time to move on to the test content chapters of this book, but be sure to keep your goal in mind. As you read, think about how you will be able to apply this information on the test. If you've already seen sample questions for the test and you have an idea of the question format and style, try to come up with questions of your own that you can answer based on what you're reading. This will give you valuable practice applying your knowledge in the same ways you can expect to on test day.

Good luck and good studying!

Data Content, Structure, and Information Governance

CURRENT TRENDS IN HEALTHCARE DATA

The role of a health information data analyst continues to evolve as the world of electronic health records matures. In this present electronic age, healthcare data (whether clinically, administratively, or financially related) is limitless. The following data trends represent the limitless opportunities of health information management (this list is not exhaustive):

- Calculation of patient wait times to be seen by a healthcare provider.
- Calculation of readmission rates (which can have a significant financial impact).
- Monitoring of complication and/or mortality rates.
- Monitoring of public health data.
- Monitoring the average length of stay.
- Analysis of patient quality scores.

Trending these data sets will tell a story upon which the healthcare entity can make important healthcare decisions (administratively, clinically, and financially) moving forward.

CURRENT HIM TRENDS

The healthcare environment is constantly changing. There are multiple opportunities for healthcare as well as the health information management (HIM) profession, and there are risks as well. A scan of the healthcare environment, and specifically how opportunities and risks are affecting the HIM profession, has identified some of the following trends: Technology advancements, cloud services, big data, mobile health, consumer control of health information, and the growth of health information exchange. Technology advancements continue to reinvent the delivery of healthcare, and in terms of how technology has affected HIM, the power of data has opened opportunities in information access and the development of new reimbursement models. Cloud services are being used to host health information applications. The existence of big Data is increasing opportunities for HIM professionals to participate in clinical informatics and/or data analysts. Mobile health services (e.g., via smartphones and tablets) are changing the landscape of healthcare delivery. Use of apps to track patient information as well as operationalize physician practices brings many opportunities for healthcare improvement as well as challenges. Consumers desire more control of their health information through online access, and as a result, health information exchange use is growing exponentially.

NCDs and LCDs
Purpose

National coverage determinations (NCDs) are published by Medicare for the purpose of noting what services or procedures will be covered by Medicare. An NCD is mandated at the national level for all fiscal intermediaries and Medicare administrative contractors (MACs) to follow. Local coverage determinations (LCDs) are established by each MAC for the purpose of establishing further guidance beyond the NCD or by providing guidance in the absence of an NCD. LCDs are applicable to the corresponding MAC's jurisdiction. NCDs and LCDs are primarily intended to provide medical necessity guidance. CMS.gov maintains a Medicare coverage database wherein one can locate NCDs and LCDs, whether they are current, retired, or proposed.

Development of NCDs by the Centers for Medicare & Medicaid Services

The Centers for Medicare & Medicaid Services develops national coverage determinations (NCDs) when there is a need to provide coverage for new healthcare technologies or procedures or when there is a need to consider an existing procedure as being beneficial for national Medicare coverage. The process of developing a new NCD takes usually between 6 and 9 months and involves assessment of the national coverage request, advisory committee reviews, staff reviews, draft decisions, public comments, and final decision implementation. Of interest, a local coverage determination (LCD) can become an NCD if approved to be adopted nationally.

Locating an NCD or LCD Online

CMS.gov/medicare-coverage-database is one of the quickest ways to locate a national coverage determination (NCD) or a local coverage determination (LCD). All NCDs and LCDs, regardless of status (e.g., active, retired, future, or proposed) are maintained in this database. Searches can be done by reviewing the alphabetic index, conducting a search for the NCD/LCD title (if known), or by searching according to geographic region. Once the desired NCD/LCD is located, either the content will be available for review immediately or one will need to select the link to the pdf file.

Following Outpatient Coding Guidelines

The Current Procedural Terminology (CPT) code set is the most widely accepted nomenclature for the reporting of physician procedures and services. It is endorsed by the U.S. Department of Health and Human Services as the nationally accepted coding standard. Each section of the CPT code book includes specific guidelines. These coding guidelines are a set of rules for coders to follow in order to appropriate interpret and report procedures and services provided in physicians' offices and/or outpatient settings. As with all coding guidelines, they promote consistency among coders and healthcare providers in the assignment of codes.

DETERMINING PRODUCTIVITY STANDARDS FOR IMPLEMENTATION OF ICD-10 CODING PRACTICES

With the recent implementation of ICD-10 coding practices beginning October 2016, there are several methods to consider for implementation pertaining to productivity standards. These methods include the following:

- Monitor the average coding time per record and trend the results. Initially, the average coding time would have increased in comparison to ICD-9 average coding times; however, over time, the average coding times in ICD-10 should begin to decrease.
- Monitor coding productivity by the case mix index (CMI). Coding productivity, for those coders working in cases with a high CMI would be longer than those with a low CMI.
- Assess the average coding time for the top 25 diagnosis-related groups (DRGs) for the designated entity.

Once all of these results are monitored and trended over a select period of time, productivity standards can be developed because these measures help to identify codes and/or DRGs for which it takes a longer period of time to complete.

ESTABLISHMENT OF CODING PRODUCTIVITY STANDARDS

The formula to calculate a coder's production is simple: Subtract the hours of noncoding tasks (also known as "downtime") from the total hours of coding tasks. Of note, noncoding tasks should include the following: education/training, system technical problems, data analysis projects, etc. Then divide the number of accounts coded by the hours spent coding. This will provide the number of accounts coded per hour. This formula can be built into database functions, available for the coder and manager to acknowledge. This formula may be easy, but there are other factors to consider when determining the coder's overall skill level. For example, quality of work or coding accuracy must be monitored, striving to reach or surpass the national standard of 95% coding accuracy.

CODING REFERENCE MATERIALS AVAILABLE IN AN ENCODER

An encoder is an electronic tool that receives diagnostic or procedural data manually entered by a coder, which then converts the data into a numerical code. An encoder is a logic-driven tool that prompts the coder through several choices/options until the appropriate code is achieved. Inevitably, the coder will encounter insufficient documentation, which leaves the coder questioning which code to assign. In these situations, the coder should access coding references to guide in his/her code selection process. These coding references are available in an encoder. The references may include the International Classification of Diseases (ICD) ICD-9 and ICD-10 Official Coding Guidelines, American Hospital Association's *Coding Clinics* dating back to the 1990s, the American Medical Association's *CPT Assistant*, Faye Brown's coding handbooks, approved medical abbreviation lists, Elsevier's *Atlas of Human Anatomy*, etc.

CODING CLINIC, CPT ASSISTANT, AND 3M NOSOLOGY

An experienced coder understands the importance of accessing reliable resources for compliant coding. *Coding Clinic, CPT Assistant*, and 3M Nosology are reliable resources frequently referenced by seasoned coders. The American Hospital Association (AHA) publishes the *Coding Clinic*, an official publication of coding guidelines and advice. The AHA Central Office works with the National Center for Health Statistics and the Centers for Medicare & Medicaid Services to maintain the integrity of the ICD-10 coding classification system. *CPT Assistant* is published and maintained by the American Medical Association as the official word on proper Current Procedural Terminology coding. 3M Nosology is a support system whose employees field coding questions and provide advice on appropriate code assignment. All three resources are valuable tools for coding professionals.

GUIDELINES FOR DATA ORGANIZATION IN EXCEL

Excel spreadsheets are an excellent tool for data organization. For the spreadsheets to contribute value to operations, it is imperative that data be organized. The following are tips on how to organize data in Excel:

- Categorize columns of similar data.
- Identify critical data with a different-colored font or apply special font (e.g., italics, bold).
- Use cell borders to designate related data.
- Avoid leading spaces in cells because the spaces can cause problems with search functionality.
- Use formulas across multiple cells for ease of calculations.
- Use data filters to locate specific data quickly.
- Use features such as wrap text to contain lengthy data fields and improve readability.
- Use numbering options across multiple cells for accounting, percentages, currency, date/time, etc., to improve readability.

DESIGNING EFFECTIVE TRAINING PLANS

The design of effective training plans should incorporate a needs assessment/analysis, design of scope and objectives, development of trainers, implementation, and evaluation. A needs assessment/analysis can be a simple process of asking questions (regarding learning needs, stakeholder involvement, and determination of desired end results) and finding answers prior to progressing forward with other steps. Once the needs assessment is complete, the learning scope and objectives should be defined along with methods of measurement. This step also involves identification of the learners, their individual skill levels, their job requirements, and the types of available resources to ensure effective training. Ideal trainers should possess leadership skills, great communication skills, and teaching abilities. Investments through time, resources, and speaking practice must be made in these trainers to ensure successful implementation. Before moving into implementation of the training, it is advisable to have a test run and then assess feedback. During the actual implementation, tracking of attendees and their pass rates of the training course should be maintained. By doing so, subsequent training can be directed to these individuals as needed. The final step is evaluation procedures through surveys to assess the effectiveness of the speakers and course materials.

TRAINING STAFF ON EHR SYSTEM

Whether implementing new electronic health record (EHR) software and providing training for all employees or providing training for new employees only, the following best practices should be incorporated into the training program: Identify each employee's computer proficiency level through testing/examinations, and then develop educational opportunities based upon identified needs. Designate team leads or superusers to whom other employees can access for assistance with computer issues. The team leads should have a high degree of computer literacy, great communication skills, teaching skills, and a positive can-do attitude. Training plans should be individually designed for each employee's job responsibilities so that, at least initially, they will only be exposed to parts of the EHR that they have a need to know. After training is completed, follow-up with each employee should be done to determine areas of improvement for future training initiatives.

MANDATES THAT PROMOTE CDI OPPORTUNITIES

Clinical documentation improvement (CDI) initiatives are not implemented because of picky health information management professionals who just desire better documentation to assist with their code assignments. Rather, there are multiple CDI mandates that are behind the push for better documentation. Federal regulations, changes in quality measures, changes in payment methodologies, and patient health and safety initiatives are all driving forces behind CDI programs. Federal mandates or initiatives include meaningful use incentive programs and recovery audit contractors. Audits by Medicare, Medicaid, and commercial insurance companies are strong catalysts behind documentation improvement because their audits can potentially change reimbursement amounts based upon poor and/or inadequate documentation. Of course, the transition to ICD-10 coding requirements has changed the documentation landscape, requiring more specific descriptions of diagnoses and/or procedures in order to assign appropriate codes. Ignoring these multiple mandates will impact financial reimbursement, as well as increased RAC activity, poor quality-of-care scores, and increased risk to patient safety.

HOSPITAL ACCREDITATION

Hospital accreditation is a peer assessment process conducted by an external agency whose primary purpose is to evaluate healthcare performance against established standards and then recommend steps to improve the delivery of healthcare. The Joint Commission is the nation's top accreditor for hospitals. The Joint Commission will award a gold seal of approval, which is internationally recognized, when a hospital meets the evidence-based standards pertaining to quality of care and patient safety. All types of hospitals (e.g., government-owned, long-term rehab, psychiatric, etc.) and treatment provided by facilities (e.g., home health, ambulatory care, etc.) after hospitalization can also achieve accreditation. In

21

addition to accreditation services, the Joint Commission promotes performance improvement to help the healthcare organization succeed even after the accreditation process is over. Additional certifications may be granted in addition to Joint Commission accreditation status, such as disease-specific care certifications, patient blood management, medication compounding, etc.

BECOMING ACCREDITED BY THE JOINT COMMISSION

Before the initial Joint Commission survey is conducted, the healthcare organization should complete the following steps, at a minimum:

- Ensure that state licensure requirements have been met.
- Ensure that the Centers for Medicare & Medicaid Services 855A application has been verified.
- Ensure that patient census requirements are met in order to provide an ample supply of records to Joint Commission surveyors.
- Request a free trial edition of Joint Commission standards.
- Request an accreditation guide.
- Apply for an accreditation survey and pay the nonrefundable fee.

Before the survey has ended, Joint Commission surveyors will schedule an exit conference to review a preliminary summary of findings. The preliminary report may be further reviewed by the Joint Commission's central office. Once the review is finalized, a final summary will be posted on the Joint Commission's extranet site. Post-survey requests for additional information may be submitted by the Joint Commission with time limits set at either 45 or 60 days. These are known as evidence of standards compliance requests. Once these are submitted by the healthcare organization, the accreditation decision will be rendered.

JOINT COMMISSION'S STANDARDS FOR HEALTH RECORDS

The Joint Commission, formerly known as the Joint Commission on Accreditation of Hospitals, promotes standards that apply to the content of health records and the timeliness pertaining to completion and authentication of those documents. The Joint Commission requires that for every patient who receives treatment at a healthcare facility, there must be a documented record of care. The documents specifically addressed by the Joint Commission pertaining to content, completion, and authentication are the history and physical, discharge summary, operative records, restraint or seclusion records, sedation and anesthesia records, medication orders, acceptable abbreviations, confidentiality agreements, organ donation records, etc. The Joint Commission assesses many functions of a hospital environment beyond health record content, and they do so every three years. With their approval, a healthcare entity can claim Joint Commission accreditation status, which attests to the public its high level of quality of care.

AHIMA'S CODE OF ETHICS

The American Health Information Management Association (AHIMA)'s code of ethics exists to guide conduct for health information professionals. These ethical standards help to promote the overall quality of healthcare. At a high level, AHIMA's code of ethics serves the following seven purposes:

1. Promote health information management (HIM) practice standards.
2. Identify HIM core values.
3. Apply broad ethical principles in support of the core values.
4. Apply ethical principles to guide decisions and actions.
5. Promote a professional behavior framework upon which ethical conflicts are addressed.
6. Promote ethical principles for accountability of HIM professionals by the public.
7. Promote mentoring of new HIM professionals.

Principles and guidelines comprise the code of ethics, promoting the following ideas:

- Advocate the patient's right to privacy and confidentiality.
- Practice HIM functions with integrity, bringing honor to the profession.
- Preserve and protect personal health information.
- Refusal to participate in unethical processes.
- Promote the HIM profession through education and research and through mentoring of HIM students.
- Promote interdisciplinary collaboration, representing the HIM profession in the collaborative efforts.

AHIMA'S STANDARDS OF ETHICAL CODING

The American Health Information Management Association (AHIMA) has issued standards pertaining to ethical coding. The standards reflect the expectations for professional coding conduct pertaining to diagnostic and procedural coding as well as the abstracting of health information. The standards are available for reference on AHIMA's web site, but an abbreviated version follows:

- Accurate, complete, and consistent coding practices are required.
- Coding compliance with regulatory guidelines is expected regarding reimbursement and data reporting.
- Documentation must support assigned codes.
- Provider queries are acceptable for the purpose of documentation clarification.
- Code assignments must not be misrepresented.
- Inappropriate assignment of codes for financial gain is prohibited.
- Continuing education to advance coding knowledge is necessary.
- Maintain the confidentiality of patient health information.

MEDICARE FRAUD AND MEDICARE ABUSE

In general, Medicare fraud can be defined as knowingly submitting false claims to obtain federal reimbursement. Examples of Medicare fraud may include billing for services not rendered, billing for services at a higher level of complexity than actually performed, billing for supplies not provided, and falsifying documentation. Committing Medicare fraud may result in civil or criminal liability, leading to imprisonment, monetary penalties, loss of credentials, and loss of Medicare funding. Medicare abuse can be defined as practices that result in unnecessary costs to the Medicare program. Examples of abuse may include billing for medically unnecessary services, charging beyond the fair market value for services or supplies, upcoding or unbundling of codes on a claim, etc. Medicare abuse violations may result in civil or criminal liability.

HEAT

In 2009, the U.S. Department of Health and Human Services and the Department of Justice created the Health Care Fraud Prevention and Enforcement Action Team (HEAT). HEAT was created for the purpose of strengthening existing programs already fighting against Medicare fraud and abuse. Some of the preexisting agencies that fight against Medicare fraud include the Comprehensive Error Rate Testing program, Medicare administrative contractors (MACs), the Recovery Audit Contractors program, and zone program integrity contractors, etc. The overall mission of HEAT is to prevent waste, fraud, and abuse of Medicare resources. HEAT governs the "Stop Medicare Fraud" website (medicare.gov/fraud), which provides information to the public on how to identify, prevent, and report fraud.

INTERNATIONAL PROFESSIONAL PRACTICES FRAMEWORK AUDITING STANDARDS

The International Professional Practices Framework is auditing guidance provided by the Institute of Internal Auditors (IIA). The four purposes of the auditing standards are to (1) guide the auditor to adherence with the framework, (2) provide a framework that promotes the value of auditing procedures, (3) establish the foundation for evaluating audit performance, and (4) cultivate improvement in organizational processes. The audit standards are divided into two categories: attribute and performance standards, with attribute standards focusing upon the organizational and auditor characteristics and performance standards focusing upon the methodology of internal auditing. All internal auditors are accountable for compliance with IIA standards.

CENTERS FOR MEDICARE & MEDICAID SERVICES PHYSICIAN COMPARE INITIATIVE

The Centers for Medicare & Medicaid Services is the creator of the Physician Compare Initiative. Physician Compare creates incentives for physicians to optimize their performance. Through the use of quality performance scores, patients/consumers can rank physicians and determine which physician to choose for services. The quality performance scores incorporate the type of delivered care and the complexity of patients that are evaluated and treated. Case mix index (CMI) values for each provider do affect Physician Compare scores; in other words, an increase in the CMI will have a positive impact upon a physician's score. Other types of data collected for providers include the number of patient deaths, complications, and diagnosis-related group assignments.

ENSURING VALID HEALTHCARE PROVIDER CREDENTIALS

Validation of physician credentials is a requirement for admitting privileges to a healthcare facility. The process of physician credentialing is performed by the medical staff office and should include the following steps:

- Collect up-to-date information on the physician applicant.
- Determine what types of information are needed about the applicant (i.e., work history, education, current curriculum vitae, board certification, state licensure, malpractice liability certificate, controlled substances certificate, etc.).
- Obtain an attestation from the physician stating that the information provided is true and complete.
- Perform a background check pertaining to education, work history, licensure, Medicare sanctions, criminal cases, etc.
- Contact peer references who can attest to the applicant's ethical work history.
- Investigate identified malpractice claims.
- Verify privileges with previous or current healthcare entities.

MONITORING THE PHYSICIAN CREDENTIALING PROCESS

Physician credentialing is a complex, ongoing, and critically important process for a healthcare entity. Once a physician is credentialed to practice at a healthcare entity, the process does not end. Credentialing must be continually monitored. One option is to purchase credentialing software packages that enhance the monitoring process. Another option is to use an Excel spreadsheet (XL SS). The XL SS should be designed to incorporate all hospitals in the system, all payers, and all providers. The deadlines for submissions of paperwork for each provider should be included. An employee should be designated to monitor the process. This employee should have the freedom to pursue completion of paperwork by applicable providers and obtain the necessary data. Both options require funding and/or staff to effectively and consistently monitor the credentialing process.

RECREDENTIALING PROCESS FOR PROVIDERS

Approximately three months prior to the expiration date of a provider's appointment to a healthcare system, the medical staff office should notify the provider of their upcoming renewal requirement. The notification should include an application for reappointment. The provider should then submit the completed reappointment application along with a copy of his/her current medical license, Drug Enforcement Administration certification, professional liability coverage, board certification status, any current disciplinary processes, health status changes, and continuing education hours. For those providers who have not actively practiced within the previous year, additional information may be requested, such as referral letters from practicing peers. If a provider's information is not sufficient for recredentialing, the burden should fall upon the provider to provide additional documents to the reviewing body for consideration.

METHODS TO KEEP DATA CLEAN

As healthcare databases grow, so does the risk of having dirty data. Methods to keep data clean should be a collaborative effort including information technology (IT) as well as health information management (HIM) personnel. IT and HIM are each instrumental in developing strong algorithms that will keep records unique and thus prevent duplicate records. IT professionals will understand how to direct data to specific locations, and HIM professionals will understand where those specific locations in the health record need to exist. The development of strong algorithms, prevention of duplicate records, and the actions of keeping data clean all fall under the umbrella of information governance. If governance is weak, then dirty data will enter the system(s) and compound IT and HIM problems downstream. The following are best practices to avoid these issues and keep data clean:

- Use advanced duplicate matching algorithms.
- Establish data integrity teams to identify dirty data and reconcile the data.
- Implement strong governance policies for ongoing data integrity.
- Implement education and training for data integrity staff.
- Implement automated data mapping, data integrity audits, and duplicate data monitoring.

IMPACT OF PATIENTS' INVOLVEMENT IN DATA INTEGRITY

With the institution of patient healthcare portals (primarily as a result of meaningful use measures mandated by the Centers for Medicare & Medicaid Services that requires providers to provide access for their patients to each patient's information), patients now have greater access to their personal health information. As a result, patients are more involved with the validation of their healthcare data. With each stage of meaningful use implementation, patients are becoming more involved. Stage 3 will provide patients with the ability to request amendments to their information online through a patient portal. Patients' involvement helps to ensure data integrity. When patients identify data inaccuracies or data anomalies, they have the ability to email the physician through the portal or click on links labeled as "medical record corrections" in order to facilitate amendments. Providers have the authority to accept or deny the amendment request according to Health Insurance Portability and Accountability Act rules.

AREAS NEEDING DATABASE MAINTENANCE

Effective database maintenance may include several areas of concern, but the following are some of the key areas that should not be overlooked. (1) Data and log file management is one of the key areas. Maintenance of these files should be checked to ensure that the files are isolated from all other database functions, that autogrowth and instant file initialization are configured correctly, and that autoshrink is not enabled. If these elements are not maintained, then the files can become fragmented and result in poorly performing queries. (2) Index file fragmentation should also be checked. Fragmentation is when there is empty or wasted space on a database page, and wasted space leads to needing more database pages, which takes up more computer disk space and initiates more complicated and time-consuming queries. (3) Corruption detection and data backups should also be checked or run during maintenance procedures. Corruption detection may identify "torn" pages in which the system was unable to complete a task due to a power failure midtask, and backups help to restore database integrity prior to a corruption event.

LEGAL HEALTH RECORD AND DESIGNATED RECORD SET

The legal health record serves the purpose of providing evidence of decisions made concerning patients' health status and treatment. It also serves the purpose of providing support for revenue requested from payers. The documentation maintained in the legal health record serves as a legal testimony surrounding patients' care. The legal health record is referenced when requests for information are received. Each healthcare entity (through a multidisciplinary approach) will determine the structure and content of their legal health record, ensuring compliance with multiple regulatory guidance. They will also determine the designated record set as it complies with the Health Insurance Portability and Accountability Act's Privacy Rule. The designated record set should include, in addition to medical information, billing records, enrollment, payment, claims, imaging (e.g., X-rays), and case management information. The designated record set is broader in content than the legal health record.

MEDICAL STAFF BYLAWS AND RULES AND REGULATIONS REGARDING LEGAL HEALTH RECORDS

The medical staff bylaws and the medical staff rules and regulations should identify the structure and content of the legal health record. Using regulations (e.g., of the Joint Commission, Office of Inspector General, Centers for Medicare & Medicaid Services, etc.) as guidance, the bylaws and rules and regulations should describe the following elements of the legal record: Definition — The collection of medical information pertaining to each patient that is treated. Maintenance — The determination of the media containing information (e.g., paper and electronic) and the integration of the media into a consolidated record. Confidentiality — The determination to comply with privacy regulations and policies. Content — The determination to meet federal and state regulations as well as accreditation requirements and to include documentation entries as soon as possible after the treatment is rendered. Documentation — The determination to follow documentation best practices and designate who is eligible to document (e.g., physicians, nurses, nurse practitioners, social workers, physical therapists, etc.). Completion, timeliness, authentication — The determination of acceptable time frames to complete the record and who is eligible to authenticate entries. Ownership — The determination of who owns the information and the parameters of securing the information on site. Retention and destruction — The determination to comply with federal and state regulations regarding the information retention. Corrections/Amendments — The determination of how documentation errors will be addressed.

27

MONITORING OF ORGANIZATIONAL NEEDS

The Code of Federal Regulations has published a standard that mandates that covered entities must have audit controls in place to monitor information systems that contain electronic patient health information. This standard does not outline the audit process, and as a result, most healthcare entities tend to react to organizational processes/needs/issues rather than proactively monitor them. Regardless of whether the audit process is reactive or proactive, the primary concern is to ensure that audits are conducted to identify organizational risks and needs. The audit process should include identification of who will be audited, which systems will be audited, the audit frequency, and reporting of audit findings in conjunction with educational efforts to correct noncompliant findings.

CHART AUDIT

When performing a chart audit, there are several steps to follow in order to issue a reliable and compliant audit. Pull from an audit plan or identify a chart topic (e.g., breast cancer) to audit. Next, identify the measures/criteria to assess. Research the audit topic or regulatory guidance to further define the audit scope, objectives, and measures. The next step would be to identify the patient population by establishing inclusion and exclusion criteria. The sample size should be defined, according to statistical frameworks, and then audit tools should be created that fit the audit scope and objectives. Collection of data would be next in the process, followed by analysis of findings and summarization of results. The audit should focus on completeness of the documentation, accuracy of the information/data, and timeliness of reports and authentication.

IMPLEMENTATION OF CORRECTIVE ACTIONS ASSOCIATED WITH AUDIT FINDINGS

As part of an internal audit process, corrective actions associated with audit findings will be recommended by the auditor to the auditee. The auditee must respond to the recommended corrective action(s) by stating how the corrective action(s) will be implemented, monitored, and deemed corrected. A time frame acknowledging the implementation date to the resolution date must be included in the auditee's response. For example, an auditee may document that the audit finding will be resolved once a 95% accuracy rate is determined through monitoring efforts and the 95% accuracy rate has been maintained for a consecutive period of six months. The auditee would then provide the corrective action plan and results to the internal audit department. The internal audit department would then be responsible for validating the resolution of errors as well as the accuracy of the provided data. The internal audit department must follow up on all open audit issues/findings with each auditee, ensuring that they are brought to resolution. This can be accomplished through automated tracking systems that alert the auditees that deadlines for resolution are approaching or have passed. If resolutions have not occurred within the initial allotted time frame, then further communication efforts should occur between the internal audit department and the auditee.

28

CLINICAL PERTINENCE REVIEWS

Clinical pertinence reviews may be conducted in a healthcare entity for the purpose of identifying the completeness and timeliness of medical record documentation and to determine actions to improve documentation practices. Clinical pertinence reviewers should be clinicians or providers of care (e.g., nurses or physicians) because they possess the clinical knowledge necessary to determine documentation inadequacies. A representative sample of records should be included in ongoing reviews, and the documentation areas to review would be as follows (at a minimum): Patient identification data, medical history, physical exam, physician orders, informed consent for treatment, progress notes of clinical observations and results of treatment, consultations, operative notes, procedure notes, final discharge diagnoses, discharge disposition, and autopsy results. Each healthcare entity should create a list of documentation areas to review to ensure compliance with federal/state regulations and/or accreditation agencies.

MANAGING AUDIT TRAILS

An audit trail can be defined as a legal record that shows all the users who have accessed a computer system, when they accessed it, and what information they accessed. Audit trails can be built to monitor any modifications, views, or deletions of data. Areas of interest that healthcare entities may monitor are the following:

- Access to health information for which the individual viewing the information has no need to know about the patient's healthcare or treatment.
- Access to information that does not correspond to the job description of the user.
- Access to high-profile records.
- Access to health information that has not been accessed recently.
- Access to fellow employees' records.
- Access to sensitive records.

Health information management and information technology (IT) professionals are responsible for managing audit trails within an EHR. Audit trails must also be retained for compliance purposes with the Health Insurance Portability and Accountability Act. Collaboration with the IT department must occur to ensure that audit trails are available for archival purposes and can be restored as needed.

MPI

The MPI is a data repository of all patients who have ever been admitted or treated at a healthcare organization. The MPI is the source of truth to reference when attempting to locate patient records. The American Hospital Association requires that certain patient information be maintained in the MPI (e.g., patient's full name, address, identifying number such as an account number and/or medical record number, and patient's birth date). Sometimes, additional information may be included such as gender, ethnicity, admission/discharge dates, and discharge disposition. Prior to the onset of the electronic health record, the MPI was managed by preparing an index card for every patient, which was maintained in an

29

alphabetical file. The MPI in the electronic world collects the same data as the old manual systems. The electronic MPI is often created by and accessible from electronic health records, and in large healthcare systems, there will most likely be an enterprise master patient index (EMPI). An EMPI links together smaller MPIs that are contained within separate systems, such as outpatient clinics, rehab facilities, and hospitals.

RETENTION REQUIREMENTS

The master patient index (MPI) is a data repository of all patients who have ever been admitted or treated at a healthcare organization. The MPI may be a manual or an electronic system. For manual systems, the index cards containing the patient information may be retained in an incorruptible format, such as microfilm or microfiche, and they may be kept on-site or off-site. For electronic indexes, the patient information should be retained in an archived state. The recommended retention period for these indexes is at least 10 years, unless state law specifies a different time frame. It is important to remember to always follow the strictest regulation. Retention time frames are influenced by federal and state laws, Medicare, and statutes of limitations.

MANAGEMENT OF PATIENT IDENTIFICATION

Accurate and consistent patient identification is an absolute necessity in today's healthcare environment, especially with an emphasis upon patient safety. Without proper patient identification, the possibilities of medication administration errors or blood transfusion administration errors can be a reality with unfortunate consequences. Therefore, a healthcare entity must have an effectively managed master patient index (MPI) or enterprise master patient index (EMPI). Some of the most common inconsistencies in MPI or EMPI platforms are duplicates and overlays. The term "duplicates" refers to one patient with multiple medical record numbers or other patient identifiers, and the term "overlays" refers to two patient records incorporated into one medical record number. Both can cause serious adverse patient events, and therefore, it is imperative that health information management departments supervise the MPI/EMPI daily.

ACCURATE PATIENT MATCHING AT REGISTRATION

Accuracy of patient identification at the time of registration is an ongoing challenge for healthcare organizations today. Collaboration between centralized and decentralized registration areas is essential to obtaining accurate patient information. A data integrity team of key information professionals should be organized to identify and correct patient identification problems between the various registration areas. Ongoing training of key staff members must be consistently applied as well. The training should emphasize the long-term effects of poor registration practices, stressing the importance of obtaining viable information, such as previous treatment at the present facility, nicknames, correct spelling of the patient's name, legal name on birth certificate, and even correct punctuation in names. Patient registration clerks should be monitored to ensure that important steps are not overlooked during registration.

TOOLS TO ADDRESS PATIENT IDENTIFICATION

Integration of various tools into the registration process can assist in the validation of patient identity. For example, biometric tools are available to scan palm veins, retinas, and fingerprints. Biometric technology scans vein patterns (whether in the palms or behind the retinas), which are unique patient identifiers. This protects against identity fraud, and enhances the registration process because it minimizes the need to reenter patient information in subsequent healthcare visits. Registrars can use valid photo IDs or driver's license to validate identity, as well as facial recognition software, and address verification cross-referenced against United States Postal Service standards.

USING BIOMETRICS DURING PATIENT REGISTRATION

Biometrics can be defined as a metrics system related to unique human characteristics. The use of biometrics during patient registration processes can reduce, or even potentially eliminate, duplicates as well as improve the accuracy of patient identity matching between multiple healthcare settings and disparate systems. Biometric software has the ability to scan fingerprints, retinas, or veins in the palms. This type of registration process would ensure reliable patient identification. In the present day, few healthcare entities use biometrics during the registration process.

CONTROL AND MANAGEMENT OF FORMS IN A FULLY ELECTRONIC HEALTH RECORD SYSTEM

In a fully electronic health record (EHR) system (meaning there are no paper records or hybrid record systems), form management and control is still a job function for health information management (HIM) professionals. Standardized documentation templates approved by a forms committee will be the structure of the EHR with patient-specific healthcare data collected in fields and mapped to other associated fields. HIM professionals would participate in the forms committee to consider new form requests and determine the appropriateness of revision requests. Forms inventory and design are a critical function of the committee. HIM professionals would be involved in the management and control of electronic forms. This would include determining record order in terms of display and indexing. When a printed record or a CD copy of the record is requested, a standardized chart order must be developed and followed. HIM professionals would be involved in the implementation of record completion standards, outlining procedures for documentation deficiencies and ensuring EHR capabilities to monitor and track documentation completion. One final step in form management and control would be for the HIM professional to determine when electronic records will be "locked" and available for "read-only" purposes.

CDI
MEANING AND PURPOSE

Clinical documentation improvement (CDI) is the process of reviewing health information for conflicting or incomplete provider documentation that fails to support the assignment of diagnostic or procedural codes. The CDI process is critically important because the health record is the primary tool used between clinicians to communicate and ensure continuity of the patient's care. Documentation should always capture the complete and accurate picture of the patient's health status and treatment, and the CDI process ensures the completeness and accuracy. CDI requires buy-in by the provider in order for it to be successful. One of the best ways to "train" each provider or to gain his/her buy-in is to demonstrate to him/her that CDI helps the provider to meet quality measures.

PROMOTING CDI OPPORTUNITIES WITH PHYSICIANS

Physicians are sometimes resistant when it comes to improving their documentation, primarily because of the belief that it entails more work for them to complete. There are, however, effective ways to promote clinical documentation improvement (CDI) among physicians. Some examples are explaining why CDI is important, explaining how CDI helps physicians meet quality guidelines, educating physicians through training sessions, providing ongoing support, and providing meaningful feedback.

COMPLETENESS OF DOCUMENTATION

The end result of incomplete documentation is twofold: (1) It impacts patient safety and (2) it impacts reimbursement. Both results require healthcare entities' attention to the completeness of documentation. Clinical documentation improvement (CDI) specialists are instrumental in a concurrent fashion for ensuring that documentation is complete. (Coders are involved retrospectively, after the patient's discharge.) With the addition of keywords or key phrases, CDI specialists and/or coders can obtain the necessary documentation to support code assignments. For example, the phrases, "manifested by" or "due to" can complete the puzzle and positively impact reimbursement amounts. Monitoring of documentation completeness can be accomplished by designing work assignments for the CDI specialists that focus upon high-risk diagnosis-related groups and/or previously identified "weak" documentation areas. Monitoring of documentation completeness by coders can be accomplished through directives or guidance that informs the coders to consider queries if cases lack sufficient documentation. For example, a query handbook should be created and provided to coders, and even auditors, for the purpose of knowing when to initiate a query.

SKILL SET AND COMPETENCIES FOR CDI SPECIALISTS

Individuals who are selected for clinical documentation improvement (CDI) specialist positions will possess either a clinical background (such as nurses with a background in case management or utilization review) or a coding background. The expectation for most healthcare entities is that individuals with a coding background must be certified as a certified coding specialist or certified professional coder, and many expect further credentials of registered health information

32

administrator or registered health information technician. For a CDI specialist position, individuals should have the following skill set and competencies:

- Knowledge of coding concepts (e.g., ICD-9, ICD-10-CM, ICD-10-PCS, and CPT).
- Knowledge of diagnosis-related group and/or ambulatory payment classification payment methodologies.
- Clinical terminology knowledge.
- Ability to analyze and comprehend providers' documentation in the electronic health record.
- Clinical knowledge pertaining to anatomy, physiology, pathophysiology, and pharmacology.
- Excellent communication skills, both verbal and written, to effectively discuss clinical cases with providers.
- Knowledge of healthcare regulations, specifically pertaining to documentation requirements and reimbursement requirements.

EFFECTIVE TRAINING FOR PROVIDERS

HEALTH DATA, CODING, AND DOCUMENTATION STANDARDS

Effective training platforms for hospital-affiliated providers should be conducted with the understanding that providers are interested in the patient-care perspective more so than the coding classification system. Physician education sessions should be provided as continuing medical education opportunities, and the goal should be to inform the provider of how effective documentation practices will affect his/her quality outcomes and pay-for-performance initiatives. Departmental medical staff meetings or quarterly staff meetings are excellent opportunities to cover documentation improvement practices. One-on-one educational sessions tend to be the best approach because the physician's own documentation practices can be highlighted. The intervention of a physician advisor in educational efforts is the most effective approach to improving documentation practices because the communication is peer-to-peer and tends to be better received. Coding roundtables are educational sessions that focus on coding, data analysis, and documentation improvement topics. This can be an opportunity for coders, clinical documentation improvement specialists, and physicians to collaborate and discuss opportunities for process change.

FEDERAL AGENCIES' DOCUMENTATION REQUIREMENTS

The Centers for Medicare & Medicaid Services Comprehensive Error Rate Testing (CERT) program provides direction pertaining to accurate and supportive medical record documentation. Providers should be familiar with these requirements, and documentation training should incorporate the requirements. One area of focus by the CERT program is insufficient documentation errors. Medical claims/bills are considered to be incorrect when documentation does not support or insufficiently supports payment for the services billed. Insufficient documentation errors may include incompleteness (e.g., unsigned, not dated, or insufficient detail of the clinical picture) and/or missing physician orders for services or procedures. Missing reports entirely, such as operative reports, would fail to support a line item on the

33

claim for the operation. Missing medication administration records would fail to support a line item on the claim for the drug reportedly administered to the patient. Illegible signatures (without a signature log to support the handwriting) would also be considered insufficient documentation. Each of these insufficient documentation examples should be expressed to providers along with examples of how to document correctly and thus prevent any potential compliance issues with CERT or other federal regulatory entities.

ROLE OF PHYSICIAN CHAMPIONS

Accurate and compliant coding is dependent upon complete and detailed documentation by the healthcare provider. The challenge for health information management professionals is convincing physicians of the importance of their role in providing valuable supportive documentation. Therefore, physician champions should be engaged in the process. Advice regarding effective documentation practices is better received by physicians from physician champions. Physician champions can stress to other physicians how efficient supportive documentation impacts the provider's own quality measures in addition to the hospital's quality measures.

USING PHYSICIAN ADVISORS IN THE CDI EDUCATIONAL PROCESS FOR OTHER PROVIDERS

In the world of clinical documentation improvement (CDI), physician advisors are essential to a successful program. The physician advisor is the liaison between the medical staff, coders, CDI specialists, and health information management personnel. The primary role of the physician advisor is to enhance other physicians' clinical understanding and provide effective means to document the clinical picture. This can be accomplished through face-to-face peer conversations to initiate an appropriate response to a query, or it can be accomplished through educational efforts aimed at improving documentation practices and how the improved documentation impacts reimbursement, physician profiling, and patient care. Not only will documentation practices improve through the involvement of a physician advisor, but also the following areas should be impacted in a positive manner: diagnosis-related group (DRG) validation, reduction in readmission rates, risk of mortality and severity of illness impact, and/or reduced DRG adjustments by external auditors.

IDEAL PHYSICIAN ADVISOR

The ideal physician advisor who advocates the clinical documentation improvement (CDI) process should possess four primary characteristics: (1) extensive clinical knowledge, (2) respect from medical staff peers, (3) effective communication skills, and (4) availability. His/Her extensive clinical knowledge should reach across all specialties. The most effective CDI program will have multiple physician advisors, with one tier of physician advisors at the top of the organizational CDI structure and another tier of service line physician advisors who can disseminate the knowledge obtained from the "senior" physician advisors. Training for the physician advisors should be extensive (lasting 40–50 hours) and should include the following

34

concepts: diagnosis-related group (DRG) structure, basic coding guidelines, reimbursement concepts, impact of code assignment upon reimbursement methodologies, and effective communication skills for interactions with clinical peers as well as coders and CDI specialists.

"IF IT ISN'T DOCUMENTED, IT HASN'T BEEN DONE"

The statement "If it isn't documented, it hasn't been done" has been a long-standing adage well known to health information professionals. Healthcare provider documentation of diagnoses and treatment rendered is the key to preventing denials, winning appeals, and preventing accusations of fraudulent activity by governmental agencies (e.g., Office of Inspector General, recovery audit contractors, etc.). The Centers for Medicare & Medicaid Services points out that clear and concise health information documentation is critical to the quality of patient care and is required for payment of services rendered. Documentation is necessary to support the medical necessity of services and to ensure compliance with regulatory requirements. Healthcare organizations must have policies and procedures in place to maintain the integrity of the health record.

PHYSICIAN DOCUMENTATION VULNERABILITIES

Physician/Provider documentation always has room for improvement, especially in a world of constantly changing healthcare regulations. The Office of Inspector General (OIG) is well aware of documentation vulnerabilities and publishes these annually in their OIG work plan. Some of the targeted areas for review of documentation are as follows: cloned notes, diagnosis specificity, and medical necessity. Cloned notes refer to previously documented notes that have been copied and pasted. A cloned note can provide inaccurate information for the current visit, which can adversely impact patient care. The vulnerability behind diagnosis specificity centers around missed opportunities for the identification of laterality, disease manifestation, and anatomical location, among others. A final vulnerability exists in terms of medical necessity that may not be supported with appropriate documentation, and subsequent payer denials may occur.

DETAILED DOCUMENTATION

With the implementation of the ICD-10 coding classification system, the expectation for more in-depth documentation became a reality. ICD-10 brought about major changes in the areas of classification axes, laterality, obstetrical trimester specificity, expansion of certain codes, and complications. ICD-10 is a multiaxial system with the primary axis of anatomy. Many diseases, however, are organized in ICD-10 based upon several axes such as etiology, site, or morphology. Laterality demands more specific documentation because many conditions (e.g., fractures, burns, ulcers) must now be identified by the affected side of the body in order to assign an accurate ICD-10 code. For any complications that arise during a pregnancy, obstetrical coding now requires the time frame of the complication (e.g., trimester). Code expansion in terms of diagnoses related to alcohol and drugs requires more specific documentation. ICD-10 codes for complications that arise postoperatively

35

have been expanded, requiring more specific documentation. All of these changes necessitate improved documentation by healthcare providers.

Access, Disclosure, Privacy, and Security

HIPAA

HIPAA is the acronym for the Health Insurance and Portability and Accountability Act. HIPAA is also known as the Privacy Rule. This act was endorsed by Congress in 2003. The Privacy Rule allows patients to have control of their own health information, all while ensuring that patients' healthcare treatment is not hindered. HIPAA defines boundaries for the use of health information and the appropriate methods to follow for disclosures. Of note, protected health information may be shared between healthcare providers without obtaining a disclosure from the patient. HIPAA does enforce accountability for protecting health information, and if violated, criminal and civil penalties do exist.

PATIENT'S RIGHTS

Under the Health Insurance Portability and Accountability Act (HIPAA) Privacy Rule, patients have rights. When patients receive healthcare services, HIPAA requires that they receive a notice of their privacy rights. This notice must describe how the healthcare entity will use/share the patient's protected health information, and how otherwise it will not be released without appropriate consent by the patient. HIPAA addresses patients' rights to access their own records and obtain a copy of their records, as well as the right to request an amendment to their health information, the right to request special privacy protection, and the right to access a minor's health information by a parent or legal guardian. Violations of patients' privacy rights may result in criminal or civil penalties.

COMPLIANCE WITH HIPAA REGULATIONS

Any covered entity is required to comply with the Health Insurance Portability and Accountability Act (HIPAA). How is a covered entity defined? A covered entity is defined as a healthcare provider, health plans, healthcare clearinghouses, and business associates (e.g., entities who transmit protected health information data or vendors who offer the services of personal health records). Compliance with HIPAA regulations means that the covered entity has taken measures to protect the privacy and security of its patients' health information.

DISCLOSURE

Disclosure can be defined as the act of sharing information. In terms of the Health Insurance Portability and Accountability Act, disclosure may mean that protected health information (PHI) has been released or transferred or that access to the PHI has been granted to a party outside of the organization who owns the information. The disclosure may happen in one of two ways: It is either an authorized disclosure or an unauthorized disclosure. An unauthorized disclosure comes with consequences or penalties.

37

SECURING HEALTH INFORMATION

Part of the Health Insurance Portability and Accountability Act (HIPAA) addresses the Security Rule. In order for providers to comply with HIPAA's Security Rule, a risk analysis must be conducted in order to identify and implement measures to ensure the security of electronic protected health information (e-PHI). The primary purpose of the risk analysis tool is to thoroughly assess potential risks and vulnerabilities to the privacy, integrity, and accessibility of a provider's e-PHI. For identified risks and vulnerabilities, a provider must initiate a risk management process. The best practice a provider can follow is to implement a continuous integrated risk analysis and management process that assesses new technologies and operations as they are initiated.

HITECH ACT

Changes were made to the Health Insurance Portability and Accountability Act (HIPAA) in 2009 for the purpose of expanding HIPAA's coverage and strengthening protection of health information. One important change was the Health Information Technology for Economic and Clinical Health (HITECH) Act, which enhanced HIPAA violation penalties. The HITECH Act is a component of the American Recovery and Reinvestment Act of 2009. Secondary to the HITECH Act, mandatory penalties now exist for willful neglect. These penalties can extend up to $250,000, with any repeated offenses extending to $1.5 million. The HITECH Act requires that all patients who are affected by a breach of their personal health information be notified of the breach.

IMPORTANCE OF PATIENT CONFIDENTIALITY

Confidentiality is a core responsibility of a healthcare organization. This ethical practice requires healthcare workers (regardless of role) to keep all patients' health information private. The basic premise behind confidentiality is trust. Trust is necessary in order for the physician-patient relationship to stay intact so that sensitive information will be shared by the patient. When a patient understands that his/her information will be kept private, he/she will be encouraged to seek out care and be open during the visit about his/her health condition. This is especially important with information pertaining to diseases of psychiatric, sexual, and/or drug/alcohol origin.

NOTIFICATION TO PATIENT AND SECRETARY OF HHS FOR A PHI BREACH

The Health Information Technology for Economic and Clinical Health (HITECH) Act of 2009 requires healthcare entities covered by Health Insurance Portability and Accountability Act (HIPAA) regulations to notify patients and the secretary of Health and Human Services of protected health information (PHI) breaches. The notification process begins with the discovery of a potential PHI violation, followed by the determination if the incident is, in fact, a violation. If a violation did occur, the healthcare entity is required to perform a risk assessment. This risk assessment must evaluate the nature and extent of the PHI involved, the unauthorized person to whom the PHI was released or who accessed the information without permission, whether or not the PHI was acquired or viewed, and the extent to which the risk has been mitigated. This risk assessment's overall purpose is to determine the probability of compromise. The level of compromise may be described as high, medium, or low, and its impact may be described as severe, moderate, or minimal. The healthcare entity bears the burden of proof to demonstrate that all notifications and the risk assessment were performed in compliance with HIPAA regulations.

CONFIDENTIALITY OF PHYSICIAN-PATIENT RELATIONSHIP

The physician-patient relationship is considered to be a contractual agreement. The patient seeks out the services of a physician, and the physician accepts the patient for treatment. During this relationship, health information is gathered and exchanged between the two parties. Trust between the physician and patient is essential for the sharing of sensitive health information. Without trust in the relationship, confidentiality would be undermined. The principle of confidentiality requires physicians to keep all patients' health information private. When a patient understands that his/her information will be kept private, he/she will be encouraged to seek out care and be open during the visit about his/her health condition. This is especially important with information pertaining to diseases of psychiatric, sexual, and/or drug/alcohol origins.

BREACH OF CONFIDENTIALITY

A healthcare privacy breach or breach of confidentiality is an inappropriate or impermissible use or disclosure of health information. This type of breach is a direct violation of the Health Insurance and Portability and Accountability Act, also known as the Privacy Rule. A breach may occur when the security or privacy of the protected health information (PHI) is compromised. If the covered entity, responsible for the breach, can demonstrate that the PHI was not viewed or that the entity has taken steps to mitigate the risk, the release may not be considered a breach. There are other exceptions to the definition of breach. In short, these breach exceptions may be described as (1) an unintentional acquisition made in good faith, (2) an inadvertent disclosure between healthcare entities, or (3) a situation in which the recipient of the PHI did not retain the information.

ENFORCEMENT OF PRIVACY AND SECURITY RULES

The Office for Civil Rights (OCR) is the governmental body responsible for the enforcement of the Privacy Rule. The OCR works in conjunction with the Department of Justice to investigate possible criminal cases of healthcare privacy breaches. The OCR investigates complaints of privacy breaches. They routinely conduct reviews of healthcare entities to determine whether they are in compliance with policies pertaining to privacy. The OCR may resolve complaints of potential privacy breaches by either determining there is no violation or determining a violation did occur that requires corrective action.

ADMINISTRATIVE, PHYSICAL, AND CLINICAL SAFEGUARDS FOR PHI

Protected health information (PHI) must be protected by administrative, physical, and technical safeguards. Administrative safeguards refer to policies and procedures that address PHI security as well as a security risk assessment and risk management plans. Physical safeguards can be in the form of facility access controls to information technology (IT) areas (e.g., badge-only access), restrictions of computer station access, use, and security, and hardware and media controls (e.g., how to properly dispose of IT media, how to backup IT media). Technical safeguards are safeguards that are integrated into IT systems to protect access to IT data. For example, individual authentication ensures that the person needing access is a valid requester.

ENCRYPTION

Encryption is a security method or control that provides protection for confidential information. Encryption applies a mathematical algorithm that scrambles data into a format that cannot be deciphered by people or computerized systems. The scrambled text is also known as ciphertext. Encryption is a reversible process, meaning that the scrambled text can be unscrambled back into its original form. When data are unscrambled, the method is referred to as decryption. In brief, encryption and decryption go hand in hand, and both functions require a cryptographic key that applies one or the other function. The cryptographic key must be kept secret in order for encryption to be fail-proof and the confidentiality of the information to be protected.

CYBERSECURITY

Cybersecurity is a method aimed at protecting information collected and maintained in the culture of information technology from cybercriminal activity. Cybersecurity is having a plan that focuses upon preventing information theft or information attacks (e.g., viruses, malware). Cybercriminals may steal health information for the purpose of maximizing health benefits from the victim's insurance plan, obtaining prescription drugs, or holding health information ransom and demanding large sums of money to return the health information to the patient or healthcare entity. The intention behind information attacks from viruses or malware may occur by a disgruntled employee or terrorists, sometimes referred to as hacktivists. Because of the numerous cyber threats increasing daily in the healthcare world, cybersecurity is an absolute necessity to protect patients' health information.

Although information technology (IT) departments contain the key individuals responsible for the security of health information, health information management (HIM) professionals should also be involved because they are knowledgeable of information workflows. Healthcare entities are wise to use their IT staff as well as HIM staff to proactively implement cybersecurity plans for the purpose of preventing cybercriminal activities. A cybersecurity plan should include a risk assessment of all software applications used by the healthcare entity. The risk assessment should look for protection gaps, and the identified vulnerable systems should be patched to close the weakness. Encryption is another vital method that should be used in the fight against cybertheft. All workstations and portable mediums should be encrypted. Encryption is effective in that it scrambles data so that they cannot be deciphered by people or electronic systems.

SECURELY TRANSFERRING EMAILS AND ELECTRONIC FILES

It is possible to transfer emails and electronic files containing protected health information (PHI) securely. There are steps involved in order to ensure the security of transmitted information. One step is to encrypt email communications. The easiest encryption method for email communications in Microsoft Outlook is to access the Trust Center under the Tools menu and select "Encrypt contents and attachments of outgoing messages." The recipient will need the sender's digital ID in order to decode the message. This same process can be accomplished through services that provide encryption keys and/or digital certificates. Files can be secured through accessing Internet sites that have an HTTPS address, and not just an HTTP address. The "S" indicates that the site is secure, which is advantageous for the use and transfer of sensitive files, such as PHI.

PASSCODES
IMPORTANCE IN PHI SECURITY

Passcodes, or passwords, are the simplest form of security for protected health information. However, they can be the easiest to crack by those with the wrong intentions. Maintaining passcodes can be frustrating for the user due to the many different passcode requirements for different systems. Healthcare entities should have effective policies and procedures (P&Ps) in place that address the requirements for passcodes. The P&Ps should incorporate at a minimum the following points to prevent passcode cracking:

- Avoid use of words written backwards.
- Avoid use of personal information.
- Use passcodes with long lengths, complex width (meaning use of symbols, and not primarily alphanumeric characters), and complex depth (e.g., passcodes that are not easily guessed).
- Use encryption.
- Instead of writing down passcodes, write down phrases that will jog the memory of the passcode.
- Change passcodes on a frequent basis.
- Lock accounts with more than three unsuccessful attempts.

DEVELOPING STRONG PASSCODES

Passcodes are one essential way to secure protected health information. They are not fail proof, however, to hackers. The following are key tips regarding strong passcodes:

- Create passwords that cannot be easily guessed.
- Change passwords frequently.
- Do not use the same password for multiple systems.
- Use a combination of capitalization, symbols, numbers, and alphabetical characters.
- Do not always capitalize the first letter of the passcode; rather, capitalize an alpha character in the middle or at the end of the passcode.

41

- Never use part of the username as part of the password.
- Use a word in its numerical equivalent of a telephone pad (e.g., "flash" would convert to 35274).
- Use two words separated by symbols.
- Use the first letter of each word in a phrase (e.g., I love McDonald's tea becomes ILMT).

MINIMUM NECESSARY

In the healthcare world of protected health information (PHI), "minimum necessary" is a common phrase. Minimum necessary can be defined as the amount of patient information that is released or accessed only when there is a legitimate need to know. When a legitimate request is validated, only the minimum necessary amount of information needed to perform a job function should be provided or accessed. It is important for healthcare employees to understand that accessing their own PHI (without going through the proper channels of a properly authorized release) is prohibited. This same prohibition applies to accessing the PHI of friends, relatives, or coworkers, unless there is a legitimate need to know. Software programs are rather sophisticated and are capable of identifying inappropriate accesses based upon an employee's name and address. For example, if an employee accesses a neighbor's PHI, the software will identify the access as a probable inappropriate access based solely upon the employee's address/locale.

ENFORCING ACCESS TO ONLY MINIMAL NECESSARY INFORMATION

Access to minimum necessary information means that healthcare employees may only have access to protected health information (PHI) for which there is a legitimate need to know. Healthcare privacy departments are tasked with ensuring that PHI is kept secure, and for those instances when the privacy has been breached, it's the privacy department's responsibility to investigate further and coordinate disciplinary action with healthcare managers. Some examples of measures that a privacy department could implement for the control of access to PHI might include the following: (1) tracking of electronic requests, (2) analysis of electronic PHI accesses, (3) investigation of verbal or emailed complaints about potential improper accesses, and (4) application of software packages aimed at identifying improper accesses.

OWNERSHIP OF MEDICAL RECORDS

The medical record is a compilation of all written, printed, or electronic information recorded by a healthcare provider as he/she communicates with the patient during the treatment or period. Because two parties are involved in the process of creating the record of collected information, the following question is raised: Who owns the medical record? The understanding in the health information management profession is that the medical record is the property of the provider who maintains it. The information maintained in the medical record can be accessed or obtained by the patient or his/her legal representative at any time upon going through the appropriate channels of releasing the information.

MEDICAL RECORD REQUEST PROCESS

Health information must be kept confidential, and the healthcare world is regulated by laws and policies that require confidentiality. In order to access patient information, there are release-of-information processes that healthcare institutions must follow to ensure that privacy is protected. An "authorization to disclose protected health information (PHI)" form must be submitted to the health information management department. The form must be completed in its entirety and must designate specifically which records to release. Requesters must present government-issued photo IDs in order to validate the release. In addition to this process, healthcare institutions are providing to patients the option of accessing their PHI through web-based portals. This can provide faster access to PHI instead of waiting up to 30 days for a release through other mediums (CDs, DVDs, paper).

WRITTEN AUTHORIZATION TO RELEASE INFORMATION

When a patient requests release of his or her health information to him- or herself or a third party, a written authorization is required. A written authorization to release information should include the following components:

- Name of the healthcare entity releasing the information.
- Name of the individual to receive the information.
- Patient's full name and other identifying data (e.g., address, date of birth).
- Purpose for needing the information.
- Type of information to be released with specified dates of service (e.g., discharge summary, operative report, etc.).
- Authorization expiration date.
- Authorization revocation statement.
- Patient's or legal representative's signature and date.

MANAGEMENT OF RELEASE OF INFORMATION ACTIVITY

To manage the release of information process requires quality control, productivity management, designation of turnaround times, and backlog management. Quality control should address internal and external requests for health information, how to track (e.g., paper versus electronic logs) and monitor requests (e.g., recording date and time received, date needed, the recipient's information, and valid authorization), how to process the requests (e.g., review the content of the requests, verification of the requester's right to access, and verification of the patient), and how to complete the requests (e.g., was the request processed in accordance with policies and procedures?). Productivity management and timeliness of request completion should be addressed to ensure continuity of care for internal requests and promote efficient turnaround times to prevent tremendous backlogs.

RESPONDING TO REQUESTS FROM LAW ENFORCEMENT OFFICIALS

The Health Insurance Portability and Accountability Act (HIPAA) allows release of protected health information to law enforcement officials without patient authorization under certain situations. It is imperative that HIPAA-covered entities follow the law when determining if such a release is permissible. It is also important to remember that state laws can trump HIPAA, so state laws must be followed as well. Expert resources should be available to assist release of information personnel when responding to law enforcement requests. References should address the type of information needed from law enforcement, how to verify law enforcement's credentials, how to confirm a case or warrant number and its association to the request, how to obtain law enforcement certification for the request, etc. Release forms should be completed in their entirety, obtaining appropriate signatures and noting the type of medical information to be released.

EFFECTS OF COURT ORDERS/SUBPOENAS ON RELEASE OF HEALTH INFORMATION

When a court order/subpoena is received in a health information management (HIM) department, it must be obeyed. The court order/subpoena will instruct the HIM director on which healthcare documents must be submitted. Upon receipt of the subpoena, it should be assessed for its validity (e.g., name and location of the court, signature of the court clerk, court seal, etc.). All court orders/subpoenas should be logged in, and HIM personnel should determine whether the requested records even exist. The requested records should be assessed for completeness, followed by copying the completed documents onto an electronic medium (e.g., a CD). A statement should be included with the copies to testify that the information is a certified copy.

HEALTH RECORD AMENDMENT

An amendment to protected health information (PHI) is an alteration of the health information upon identification of a documentation error. The amendment may come in the form of a deletion, addition, modification, late entry, resequencing, and/or reassignment. Removing information from a record or adding additional information may be necessary to right the error. Retracting information may correct information that is invalid or incorrect. A late entry may provide vital information that affects reimbursement because it may provide documentation to support a code assignment. Reassignment may move information from one source document to another, more accurate episode of care. It is important to note that for deletion cases, the PHI should never be entirely deleted from the record, but rather the information should be hidden from the general view.

PATIENT'S RIGHT TO PHI AMENDMENTS

The Health Insurance Portability and Accountability Act (HIPAA) provides patients with the right to request an amendment of their protected health information (PHI). HIPAA does limit the entity's right to deny an amendment. Denial of amendment requests can only occur if the PHI was not created by that particular entity or if the PHI is correct and not in error. If an amendment request is approved and completed, it is the entity's responsibility to pass along the revised information to involved healthcare providers. Revisions/amendments of PHI may need to occur in electronic or paper formats, and for the electronic changes, collaborative efforts with IT may be necessary to implement the changes. In the case of psychiatric amendment requests, the psychiatric provider of care must approve the request before the amendment can be addressed.

44

HEALTHCARE STAFF'S KNOWLEDGE ABOUT PRIVACY AND CONFIDENTIALITY ISSUES

The Health Insurance Portability and Accountability Act (HIPAA), also known as the Privacy Rule, is a federal law. It is important for healthcare staff to understand their role in ensuring compliance with this law. Compliance with HIPAA is not the responsibility of physicians or healthcare administrative staff only. Protecting the privacy and security of health information is the responsibility of all healthcare workers, whether they serve in a clinical role or a nonclinical role. Therefore, all healthcare staff must be knowledgeable of the following (at a minimum): (1) what information is protected, (2) when it is appropriate to disclose protected health information, (3) the types of healthcare information that are considered sensitive with more strict regulations, (4) the types of penalties (criminal and civil) for confidentiality breaches, and (5) the consequences of breaches to include disciplinary action, loss of job, and lawsuits.

> **Review Video: Confidentiality**
> Visit mometrix.com/academy and enter code: 250384

DATA ARCHIVE AND BACKUP POLICY

When developing a data archive and backup policy, a healthcare entity (usually collaboration between each healthcare department and the information technology [IT] department) must decide if archived files will be stored together with the backup files. Most healthcare entities choose to separate the two files. Backup files may be saved to local drives or sent to remote servers. This decision will depend on the speed of the network, the size of the drive or server, and the healthcare entity's security requirements. Backup to a local drive has the benefits of higher reliability and higher security because data are not transferred throughout the network. Regarding archived files, a dedicated server is a good choice, but the cost may not be justified if it is only designated for one department in the healthcare system. Furthermore, archived files are, in essence, a backup snapshot that overwrites a previous snapshot. Because earlier snapshots are overridden by the most recent snapshot, it is recommended that multiple backup snapshots be archived to prevent loss of data in the event of a system failure. Archival of multiple snapshots may save the day in the case of file corruptions because IT can backtrack to precorruption snapshots and start over with the old data.

RETRIEVING ARCHIVED MEDICAL INFORMATION

As patient health information ages and electronic storage space becomes limited, it is necessary for healthcare institutions to archive the information in accordance with Federal and state regulatory retention guidance. Once the data are archived, they cannot be changed or deleted prior to the retention guidance, and this principle is known as immutability. The immutability of data ensures the authenticity of the data from a legal perspective. Because large amounts of archived data will need to be maintained for potentially a long period of time, storage space can be of concern; however, technology allows for intelligent compression of the data, and this process reduces the amount of storage space. In order to locate archived medical

45

information, effective indexing and searching techniques must be used. Security of the medical information data must also be incorporated into the archival process.

HEALTHCARE RETENTION POLICIES

Healthcare retention policies must be a requirement for healthcare providers. A formal plan of retention or a record retention schedule should be developed and maintained by the health information management director. This plan should define active and inactive records/information. Statutes of limitations should be addressed in the policies as well as the requirements set forth by the federal Conditions of Participation, the *Federal Register*, the Joint Commission, state regulations, and American Health Information Management Association regulations. Record retention policies should outline the method of destruction or archiving of health information in its various mediums.

REGULATORY BODIES PROVIDING GUIDANCE FOR RETENTION OF HEALTHCARE INFORMATION

Retention of healthcare information or medical records is regulated by various external agencies. The federal Conditions of Participation is one of the most prominent regulations governing this aspect of health information. The *Federal Register* is another source that provides guidance pertaining to retention requirements. State-specific requirements exist as well. The Joint Commission, a healthcare accrediting body, weighs in on retention requirements, as does the American Health Information Management Association (AHIMA). Among federal, state, Joint Commission, and AHIMA's guidance, each healthcare entity must follow the guidance that is more restrictive. Retention hinges upon whether records are deemed active or inactive, with "active" meaning the information is still being consulted on a regular basis, and "inactive" meaning the information is rarely accessed.

CUSTODIAN OF EHRS

The custodian of the electronic health record (EHR) will be the health information management (HIM) professional. This person will have been designated as the one responsible for the care, custody, and control of the health records for patients who have received service at that healthcare entity. This HIM manager will be considered to be the custodian of the EHR in collaboration with information technology (IT) personnel because IT is instrumental in the technical infrastructure of the EHR. This HIM person will have been authorized to certify EHRs as the legal health record after inspection of the documents and after duplication of the EHR. This HIM person may also be required to testify in court as to the validity of the EHR. Certification of EHR documents attests that the copy provided to a court of law is an exact duplicate of the original.

REPORTING PRIVACY VIOLATIONS INTERNALLY

When an employee suspects a privacy violation, he/she should immediately alert his/her manager. If this is not an appropriate option (e.g., the manager may be the violator), the privacy officer and/or corporate compliance officer (CCO) should be notified through email or by calling the healthcare entity's employee compliance hotline. An option to report a suspected privacy violation anonymously must be made available to employees, such as by a compliance hotline. CCOs or privacy officers will further investigate the suspected violations through interviews, interrogations, and computer analysis. The determination to proceed with seeking the advice of legal counsel will be made, and the reporting of violations may be necessary depending upon the severity of the violation. Disciplinary action, up to and including termination of the violator's employment, may be an appropriate course of action.

REPORTING HEALTHCARE PRIVACY VIOLATIONS TO REGULATORY BODIES

Anyone can file a privacy or security violation complaint with the Office for Civil Rights (OCR). The complainant, as mentioned, can be anyone — a healthcare employee who works for the entity at which the violation has allegedly occurred or someone not affiliated with the healthcare entity. The complaint can be filed in writing, via fax, through email, or via the OCR portal. When filing the complaint, the following information should be provided: name of the complainant, contact information, and details of the suspected violation. After receiving the complaint, the OCR will investigate further and will only take action if it is determined that rights were violated and the complaint was filed within 180 days of its occurrence. The OCR will issue a letter describing its investigation, and it may issue corrective action for the healthcare entity or impose civil monetary penalties.

Data Analytics and Use

COLLECTING DATA FOR QUALITY REPORTING

Quality reporting is a function used by healthcare entities to promote quality improvement initiatives, such as core measures, meaningful use measures, physician quality reporting initiatives, etc. For quality reporting methods to be reliable, it is important to ensure that the data collected to support the quality reporting methods are valid and useful. Factors to consider when collecting data are as follows:

- Determine what information needs to be collected.
- Determine what are the information sources.
- Determine how the information will be collected.
- Determine how much information should be collected.
- Determine timelines to meet quality reporting deadlines.

Once these factors are established, it is then important to determine how the data will be used to construct or calculate the quality measures. To construct or calculate quality measures, the following steps should be done:

1. Determine the definition of each measure.
2. Define eligibility in the patient population.
3. Establish the numerator and the denominator.
4. To obtain the performance percentage, divide the numerator by the denominator.

DATA ABSTRACTION FROM MEDICAL RECORDS

Abstracting is the process of gleaning pertinent information from the medical record upon patient discharge. For healthcare entities that are still using paper records, data can be collected in two ways: (1) by manually completing a paper abstract or (2) by manually keying in the information into a computerized database. More commonly in today's healthcare environment, automated abstracting is the common practice. Clinical abstracting software automates and streamlines the capture of pertinent data and is designed to easily analyze and generate reports of coded data, clinical data, research data, and reimbursement data. Efficient abstracting software aids in reducing billing delays. Encoders and computer-assisted coding (CAC) are instrumental in the automated abstracting process. CAC automatically mines for data through its natural language processing tool, which is capable of identifying specific data from a patient's chart, and afterwards it completes predefined templates designated by the healthcare entity.

PURPOSE

The primary reason to abstract healthcare data is to generate meaningful reports reflecting diagnoses encountered and treatment provided. As healthcare moves forward, the concept of "big data" becomes more relevant. Data provide a historical healthcare picture, the present-day situation, and predict future performance models. The demands of regulatory agencies necessitate data abstraction and analysis. Meaningful use, population health, algorithms related to clinical informatics and reimbursement models, and as healthcare reform are some examples of such forces that push for data dependence and reliability. It is imperative that health information management (HIM) professionals be subject-matter experts of healthcare data abstraction and analysis. HIM professionals are the most knowledgeable when it comes to knowing how to gather meaningful data and how to manipulate them through electronic health record technology and reporting tools.

The purpose of data abstraction is to extract pertinent information from the medical record for multiple reasons. Standard data that should always be abstracted for statistical reasons (e.g., case mix index), reporting reasons, and compliance reasons are as follows: admit type (e.g., inpatient, outpatient, observation), admission source (e.g., transfer from another healthcare facility, emergency, scheduled), referring institution (e.g., skilled nursing facility, physician's office), discharge status (e.g., expired, alive), discharge destination (e.g., home, skilled nursing facility, hospice), cause of death (e.g., stroke, cancer, myocardial infarction), gestational age (e.g., 39 weeks), birth weight (e.g., 3500 g), deceased date/time, admitting physician, attending physician, and consulting physicians. Data abstraction can be accomplished manually (even though this is pretty much a thing of the past) or through the use of a health information management computer-assisted coding system.

REVIEWING ACCURACY OF ABSTRACTED HEALTH DATA

In hospitals, medical record coders will be the individuals responsible for abstracting health data as part of the coding process. Coding auditors will then review the accuracy of the abstracted data. Review criteria must be established for the accuracy reviews to occur. The criteria may include checking for the accuracy of admission/discharge dates, discharge disposition codes, the patient's gender, the patient's age, and patient type (inpatient/outpatient). In addition to abstracted patient-specific data, other reviews may focus upon the accuracy of the attending physician name, consulting physician name(s), surgeon name(s), dates of consults and procedures, and accuracy of physician queries. When reviewing the accuracy of physician queries, one would need to assess if the query was even needed, if the correct query form was used, and if the correct physician was queried. When inaccuracies are discovered, coders should be notified of recommended changes to the abstracted data. Upon review of the recommendations, the coder can either agree or appeal. If appealed, a third review may be necessary by management to determine the correct data to abstract.

DATABASE DESIGN SKILLS

Database design in today's health information market is a critical step needed to manage electronic health data. To be successful in database design, several skills are necessary. Some of these skills will include, at a minimum, the following:

- Data analysis.
- Data retrieval and reporting.
- Ability to partition data.
- Ability to read data dictionaries.
- Access, Excel, and Structured Query Language (SQL) knowledge.
- Understanding of database security and access control.
- Ability to network databases.
- Understanding of if/then formulas.
- Ability to diagram and map out/flowchart database logic.
- Ability to troubleshoot error messages.
- Ability to change database designs when needed.
- Understanding of indexing data to enhance query requests.
- Understanding of backup procedures and restoration of data.
- Ability to ensure data quality.

Of these recognized skills, fluency in SQL commands is the most important. SQL commands are used to create, manipulate, and modify data, which is the core of database design and management.

DATA DICTIONARY

FUNCTION

A data dictionary can be defined as a tool used by healthcare organizations for the purpose of ensuring accurate data collection. In order for data to be reliable and usable, all users and owners of the data must understand/interpret their meaning based upon the same source of truth — a data dictionary. According to a "Practice Brief" issued forth by the American Health Information Management Association, "standardizing data enhances interoperability across systems," and data dictionaries promote this necessary standardization. A data dictionary should describe the meaning of each data element. For example, (1) naming conventions must match between systems, (2) definition of data elements must be explained, (3) field lengths of data elements should match between systems, (4) data types (e.g., alpha, numeric, etc.) should match between systems, and (5) data frequency (e.g., monthly, annually, etc.) should match between systems. To reiterate, the primary goal of a data dictionary is to achieve standardization of data elements between various systems.

BENEFITS

The purpose of a data dictionary is to ensure and/or promote data integrity. It provides a clearer understanding of all data elements, aids in locating data, and promotes overall good data management. In addition to these attributes of an effective data dictionary, there are other benefits, as follows:

- Improved data quality.
- Improved data reliability.
- Improved data control.
- Reduced duplication of data.
- Data consistency.
- Effective and efficient data analysis.
- Better decisions secondary to better data.
- Improved standardization.

BUILDING A DATA DICTIONARY IN MICROSOFT ACCESS

A data dictionary will be comprised of field names, field types, tables, and reports. Microsoft Access is an excellent database tool to use in the healthcare setting. To create a data dictionary, there will need to be a database containing the information needed to build the dictionary. The first step would be to open the appropriate database in Access, followed by clicking the "Database tools" tab and the "Database documenter." Next, select the table(s) to include in the dictionary and the queries to include. The "Options" button will allow for selection of the various attributes needed to meet the unique characteristics of the desired data dictionary. If desired, a report can be run after these choices are made and the dictionary is built, and the report can be saved to an Excel file through the "Export" dialog box. Of note, the steps may vary depending upon the version of Microsoft Access being used. Data dictionaries may also be built in other platforms, such as SQL or Oracle.

DATA ANALYSIS TOOLS

In the healthcare marketplace, there are many data analysis software packages available for purchase. In Excel, PivotTables are an excellent tool to summarize data into categories and filter that data in various meaningful ways. Excel offers the option of working with frequency tables, which provide a means of summarizing data based upon how often each data element occurs. Excel provides a means of displaying data in an effective manner through the use of tables and charts. In addition to Excel, healthcare data analysts can use predictive modeling to analyze historical data for the purpose of identifying patterns upon which to base future decisions. Descriptive and inferential statistics are two more types of data analysis, which can be meaningful to a healthcare organization. Types of descriptive and inferential statistics are as follows: central tendency, mean (e.g., geometric length of stay) or average (e.g., average length of stay), median, mode, percentiles, range, standard deviation, and confidence intervals.

QUANTITATIVE ANALYSIS OF MEDICAL RECORDS
PURPOSE

Quantitative analysis of medical records or electronic health record information is performed by health information personnel. The purpose of quantitative analysis is to identify documentation areas that are incomplete or inaccurate. Examples of

51

documentation deficiencies may be a missing signature on a dictated history and physical report or a progress note, or a missing report entirely such as a discharge summary. Regulatory guidance regarding documentation requirements provide the basis for identifying deficiencies, and health information management departments should always compose a deficiency list based upon external regulations as well as bylaws and medical staff rules and regulations.

COMPONENTS

Quantitative analysis of medical records or electronic health record information is the process of identifying documentation deficiencies. The identified deficiencies must be resolved by the healthcare provider within a time frame of up to 30 days depending upon the type of deficiency. When analyzing for deficiencies, there are certain basic components that must be addressed, as follows: correct patient identification on each form, presence of all required reports (as mandated by The Joint Commission, hospital bylaws, medical staff rules and regulations, Centers for Medicare & Medicaid Services regulations, etc.), and authentication on all entries.

QUALITATIVE ANALYSIS OF MEDICAL RECORDS
PURPOSE

Qualitative analysis of medical records or health information is the process of identifying deficiencies pertaining to incomplete or inaccurate documentation. The health information management professional analyzing the documentation must understand disease processes in order to identify the deficiencies. For example, a provider may have failed to include the type of congestive heart failure (diastolic versus systolic), which is relevant information when assigning diagnostic codes. The healthcare provider can be queried to obtain clarification or further information, and it is the healthcare provider who makes the final decision that documentation is incomplete or inaccurate. Effective qualitative analysis will, in some cases, impact reimbursement as well as the quality of patient care.

COMPONENTS

The components of qualitative analysis should include review of the following: (1) Diagnostic statements for completeness (e.g., the final diagnoses in the discharge summary should include the principal diagnosis, complications, and any comorbidities that affect the hospitalization). (2) Consistency in documentation by all providers so that conflicting information is avoided (e.g., physician orders for drugs should match the medication administration record). (3) Justification for medical necessity throughout the patient's hospitalization (e.g., documentation must justify the course of the patient's entire stay). Presence of informed consent and/or consent to treatment (e.g., description of planned operation or description of potential medication side effects).

DATA ANOMALIES
IDENTIFICATION

In the era of big data, it is vitally important to analyze data for anomalies. Anomalies are those unusual occurrences in which the actual result differs from the expected results. Targeted areas for anomaly analysis should include moving averages, trend analysis, statistical control analysis, and basic statistical analysis. Moving averages can be established to assess a set of data points (e.g., every 4 weeks, quarterly) to identify averages in which their trends are skewed significantly. With significant skewing and/or identified outliers, potential data anomalies may be indicated. Trend analysis is a key function to identify variations of current performance in comparison to past performances, and it may identify data anomalies in need of further investigation. Basic statistical analysis pertaining to standard deviations from the center of distribution is another valuable technique of anomaly analysis.

RESOLVING ANOMALIES

Data anomalies and/or data errors are all too common in healthcare documentation practices. Data integrity is critical to the promotion of patient safety, quality of care, and efficiency. To ensure data integrity and eliminate risks associated with data anomalies, it is imperative for a healthcare organization to prove that data are authentic, timely, accurate, and complete. Documentation policies and procedures should be created and implemented to comply with regulatory and accreditation guidance. The policies should be enforced and monitored by governance controls. Templates and scripts are one way to promote data integrity. The templates and scripts can be designed to discourage copying and pasting notes by limiting field size and limiting text fields. Data models can be used to promote data integrity because they set parameters for the behavior of data and the communication between electronic health record systems. Standardization of data definitions and the structure of data fields will also limit the use of free text. Naming conventions, abbreviations, and acronyms should be standardized as another means of resolving data errors.

UNCOVERING FAILED PATIENT MERGES

Through the use of effective data analytics, it is possible for health information management professionals to identify instances wherein patient information may not have merged into one electronic record. For example, if an information merge from disparate systems fails, patient information is then kept isolated from a consolidated record. This scenario is a risk to the patient's health and safety. A data analytics program can be developed through Excel PivotTables and/or Access queries to search the database for the unidentified records. For example, newborns are commonly referenced as "Baby Girl" or "Baby Boy" at birth. Their names should be updated to their given name at a future time, but if this process is not carried out, then their information could potentially never be matched with future healthcare occurrences. Therefore, data analytics should be used to query for the generic names and their possible matches with legal names through matching patient identifiers, such as Social Security numbers.

PROBLEMS WITH COPY AND PASTE FUNCTION IN EHRS

The copy and paste functionality is an option available in an electronic health record (EHR). Although it offers providers a fast and easy way to document, it also fosters documentation errors. In an EHR, to copy and paste means to reuse all or part of documented text from one part of the record to another part of the record. Documentation errors are of concern because tracking the progress of the patient's condition can be hard to decipher. This may alert auditors to potential noncompliance issues and result in over- and/or under-reimbursement amounts. A reader may misinterpret the extent of a diagnosis if text is copied and pasted over and over throughout the record. For example, documentation of a minor hematoma copied and pasted multiple times may lead the reader/coder to think it is more complex and being consistently monitored throughout the stay, when in reality it was only noted at the time of admission with no further attention being given to it. The coder may then assign a more complex code, resulting in a noncompliant diagnosis-related group assignment. This carelessness of duplicate documentation must be vetted by the healthcare entity, and thorough policies and procedures should be developed to control the process.

LIMITING COPY FUNCTIONALITY OF MEDICAL INFORMATION

The use of copy functionality in an electronic health record is frequently used to ease the physician's burden of redocumenting the same medical information (i.e., past medical history) repeatedly. Copy functionality, or duplication of information, can be hazardous to patients' health because it can be misleading, inaccurate, and inconsistent and it can increase the risk for medical errors. Therefore, it is necessary for healthcare entities to identify ways to limit the use of copy functionality. Such limitation measures may include

- Identification of copied information as originating from a different source.
- Data transfer restrictions established to prevent copying and pasting information from other sources.
- Restrictions established that prevent one author reusing another author's information.
- Implementation of methods aimed at monitoring providers' copying and pasting actions.
- Implementation of methods aimed at monitoring audit trails.

EXCEL SKILLS FOR DATA ANALYTICS THAT HIM PROFESSIONALS SHOULD ATTAIN

In the current state of the health information management (HIM) environment, proficiency in data analytics is essential. HIM professionals must know how to analyze data, and an important tool in data analysis is Excel. An Excel spreadsheet is not just a tool to collect data; it is also a tool to tell a story with the data that allows decisions to be made. An in-depth knowledge of Excel promotes ease and efficiency of work practices. The following are tasks that HIM professionals and/or data analysts should be proficient in:

- Data reconciliation through the VLOOKUP function.
- Conditional formatting of cells to control data input.
- Pivot tables and pivot graphs/charts (to include trending and slicer options).
- Data filtering options.
- Data sorting functionality.

- Mathematical and/or statistical formula options.
- Removal of duplicate data functionality.

HEALTHCARE INTELLIGENCE

"Healthcare intelligence" is the coined phrase for the process of organizing and analyzing data at a deeper level. Healthcare intelligence focuses on transforming raw clinical data into meaningful information that can be used for numerous healthcare purposes. The data analysis component of healthcare intelligence processes historical as well as current data, and then analysts can use the results in predictive analysis. Through intelligence methodologies, analysts, also known as clinical informaticists, can drill down through exponential volumes of data to identify even the smallest of errors or compliance issues. In addition to clinical data collected in electronic health records, other types of data privy to healthcare intelligence analysis may include financial data, inventory data, and utility data. The primary objective of healthcare intelligence is to improve the continuity of care and improve clinical outcomes for patients.

COLLECTING AND ANALYZING DATA FOR SUBMISSION TO HEALTHCARE REGISTRIES

Prior to the submission of data to a healthcare registry, it is necessary to the healthcare entity to collect and analyze data. The first step in the collection and analysis process is to determine why the data are being collected. Is it for internal purposes such as quality improvement, or is it a state requirement? The next step would be to determine who will collect and analyze the data, what the data will represent, when the data will be collected and analyzed, where the data will be maintained, and how the data will be collected and analyzed. The analysis component must validate the accuracy of the data. A process must be implemented to address any data inconsistencies discovered in the process. Once these steps are planned, implemented, and tested, then the data may be submitted to healthcare registries.

DISEASE AND IMMUNIZATION REGISTRIES

A disease and immunization registry is a tool that tracks the clinical outcomes and associated treatments of a designated patient population. These registries typically house data pertaining to chronic diseases such as diabetes, heart disease, and lung disease. Through the collection of data in these registries, the quality of patient care can be improved because ultimately the data can portray opportunities for enhanced healthcare and improved patient outcomes. Health information management professionals should consider registry compatibility when selecting an electronic health record (EHR) platform and upgrading to a new EHR. It is advised to purchase and implement an EHR system that allows the healthcare entity the opportunity to create internal registries unique to their healthcare landscape. A beneficial registry will offer healthcare entities the ability to produce disease-specific reports, progress reports, exception reports, and patient population reports.

55

FUTURE OF HEALTHCARE DATA INTEGRATION

In healthcare, data originates in multiple "silos" making it necessary for entities to centralize the data for electronic health record purposes; however, the process of data aggregation can be difficult due to complex data sources. Many healthcare entities resort to the process of extract, transform, and load (ETL) for data aggregation. The ETL process involves writing scripts to transform existing data into supported formats. Although the ETL process may bring data together, it does not solve the root problem of disconnected data sources. It is imperative that moving forward, healthcare entities find ways to improve the flow of health information for continuity of patient care. This means health information disparate systems must be linked while maintaining privacy and security. This desired concept moves healthcare entities toward an interoperable information space that enables semantic integration across platforms, regardless of whether the database is an enterprise electronic health record, an isolated departmental data source, or a practice management system. Semantic technology improvements, mapping strategies, and data normalization will be the future of healthcare data integration.

COMMON REPORTS USED FOR DATA ANALYTICS

In the health information field, data analytics is a common daily task. Obtaining meaningful and relevant data is the primary objective. The following are examples of common data analytical reports generated by health information professionals:

- Calculation of readmission rates
- Case mix index analysis
- Monitoring of complication or comorbidity/major complication or comorbidity rates.
- Monitoring of mortality rates.
- Monitoring data dictionary statistics.
- Trending inpatient and outpatient coding accuracy rates.
- Trending average length of stay.
- Monitoring financial impact of diagnosis-related group and/or ambulatory payment classification changes.
- Monitoring adverse drug reactions.
- Monitoring recovery audit contractor appeals.
- Monitoring payer denials.

With more and more healthcare entities understanding the power of data analysis, the possibilities for additional data monitoring and trending are endless.

PRESENTATION OF DATA ANALYSIS RESULTS

Once data are compiled and interpreted, the findings must be presented in practical, easy-to-understand terms. To begin the presentation, the reviewer should introduce the purpose of the study, the department studied, and the population studied. The introduction should also include how the data were gathered, the sources of the data, the time frame of data collection, and the names of those who conducted the study. An interpretation section should follow the introduction. Interpretation

56

means to determine the meaning and the significance of the data analysis. Some questions for consideration might be: Why did the results turn out the way they did? What are some possible explanations of the data results? Next, a judgment should be made regarding the data results. In other words, do the results have a positive or negative impact and why? What is good or bad about the results? Finally, recommendations should be made in the presentation of data analysis. What should be accomplished as a result of the data analysis, and how will the stakeholders' responsibilities be affected?

DATA PRESENTATION

Data alone do not necessarily tell a story or show trends or even suggest successes or failures. Compiling data and then analyzing them is one step in the right direction toward providing insight into successes and/or failures and subsequently assist in making decisions. After the data have been synthesized, the next step is to present the information, usually to management or administration. Excel is an excellent tool that can extract significance from big data, specifically through PivotTable functionality. Charts and graphs can subsequently be generated from PivotTable functions and then linked into PowerPoint presentations or SharePoint dashboards. When creating visual presentations, determine the main objective that needs to be represented to the viewer. There should always be a singular point to make about each slide so that the viewer's comprehension or insight into the data's meaning will be quickly attained.

Techniques to effectively communicate the meaning of data include the following:

- Simplify the focus.
- Be methodical and clear with the data presentation.
- Eliminate distractions.
- Choose the type of chart/graph that is impactful to the viewer (e.g., bar, pie, line graphs, etc.).
- Replace text with visuals.

FUNCTIONALITY OF PIVOTTABLES AND PIVOTCHARTS IN EXCEL

In Excel, PivotTables are an excellent tool to summarize data into categories and filter the data in various meaningful ways. A health information management (HIM) analyst whose responsibility may be data collection and data comparison will find that PivotTables make data collection and comparison easier to complete. Once data are categorized and filtered within a PivotTable, a PivotChart can be created for presentation purposes. To create the PivotChart, the HIM data analyst must select data from the PivotTable, choose the best chart style (e.g., bar, column) to represent that data, and generate the chart. The PivotTable and PivotCharts can be manipulated on a prescribed timetable (e.g., for quarterly reporting purposes) with the addition of new data.

PRESENTING CODING COMPLIANCE AUDIT DATA TO THE ADMINISTRATION

In healthcare entities, coding compliance audit data pertaining to accuracy, productivity, and net financial impact will be of interest to administrators on a quarterly basis. PowerPoint slides representing these three components are best displayed as follows: Use visual graphs rather than words to communicate pertinent information. For coding accuracy, use trending bar graphs instead of stacked columns or pie charts. Trending bar graphs will provide administrators with a snapshot of how accuracy rates fluctuate from month to month. The trending bar graph should include the expected benchmark standard (e.g., 95%) graph line as well as inpatient and outpatient coding accuracy rates that may trend above or below the benchmark percentage. For productivity rates, trending should be used with explanations included as to any decrease in volume (e.g., vacations, training, vacancies, etc.). The net financial impact should be represented from two perspectives: the current quarterly monetary value (positive or negative) and the year-to-date monetary value. These three components of coding compliance audit activities may be used for other purposes, such as cost-benefit analyses, cost justification for additional staff, etc.

DATA DASHBOARDS

Data dashboards are becoming more frequently created and implemented in the healthcare environment. Dashboards are a snapshot reflection of analyzed data in various formats. Dashboards provide a quick glance (usually to the administration) of key performance indicators (KPIs) relevant to various processes (i.e., coding accuracy, case mix index trending, admission/discharge stats, etc.). The dashboard is usually available on a secured web page linked to a database (Access or Excel), and the supporting database is typically supplied with data by multiple departments who contribute information pertaining to their workflow processes and outcomes. The benefits of data dashboards are as follows:

- Ability to quickly visualize graphics of KPIs.
- Ability to identify trends associated with financial impact (typically negative). Ability to measure efficiencies and inefficiencies.
- Ability to make informed decisions.
- Ability to identify data outliers.

COMPUTING PERCENTAGES

Percentages are widely used in healthcare statistics; therefore, it is essential to know how to compute percentages. A percentage is defined as the whole divided into one hundred parts. A percentage can be misleading to organizational stakeholders if the total volume (or whole) is 20 or fewer. Therefore, it may be necessary to report only when the volume is greater than 20, which may mean quarterly or annual reporting. A percentage can be computed when a fraction is converted into units of 100. For example, if the fraction is 3/4, then the percentage is computed by dividing 3 by 4, resulting in a decimal of 0.75, which is then converted into a percentage by moving the decimal two places to the right and adding the percent sign (%). For decimal results that are lengthy (e.g., more than 2

58

decimal places), the healthcare entity/department should have a policy that designates the number of decimal places to round to (e.g., 21.456% would round to 21.5%). Once a percentage is calculated, it may be referred to as a rate. In health information management practices, rates are a common calculation, such as death rates, birth rates, readmission rates, etc. It is important to ensure that percent calculations are computed correctly because it can be easy to misrepresent the true picture.

CALCULATION OF MORTALITY RATES

Death rates, also known as mortality rates, are important information in healthcare because they can represent the quality of health services. Death rates are represented in percentages and represent the number of inpatient hospitalizations that ended in death. Dead on arrival cases, abortions (whether therapeutic or spontaneous), and patients who expire in the emergency room (without an order for admission to the hospital) are not included in the rate.

The following are various death rates that can be calculated:

- Gross death rate (number of deaths of inpatients in a period/number of discharges [including deaths] in the same period).
- Net death rate (total number of deaths of inpatients — deaths occurring less than 48 hours from admission/total number of discharges [including deaths] — deaths occurring less than 48 hours from admission)
- Anesthesia death rate (defined as a death occurring while the patient is under anesthesia or caused by anesthetic agents).
- Postoperative death rate (defined as deaths occurring within 10 days after surgery).
- Maternal death rate.
- Neonatal death rate.

LENGTH-OF-STAY CALCULATIONS

Length of stay refers to the number of days a patient is designated as an inpatient — from the date of admission until the date of discharge. This calculation is monitored daily by healthcare entities because it helps to evaluate and manage hospital resources. To compute the length of stay, the date of admission is subtracted from the date of discharge. For example, if a patient was admission on February 2 and then discharged on February 9, the length of stay would be 7 days. If the patient is admitted and discharged the same day, the length of stay is counted as 1 day. The average length of stay (ALOS) is a rate consistently monitored by healthcare entities. The ALOS rate is calculated by dividing the total length of stay (also known as discharge days) by the total discharges. For example, 1,500 patients were discharged during the month of February. The combined length of stay for these patients was 7,552 days. The ALOS rate would be calculated as follows: 7,552/1,500 = 5.03 or rounded to 5 days.

MEASURES OF CENTRAL TENDENCY

In statistical analysis, central tendency is known as a single measure that determines the center or middle value of a data set. There are three measures of central tendency: the mean, median, and mode. Health information management professionals should be familiar with these three measures because they are commonly used in healthcare statistics. The mean is the average of the numerical values in a data set. To calculate the mean, the numerical values are summed and then divided by the number of values in the data set. For example, the mean of 2 + 3 + 6 + 4 = 15/4 = 3.75. The median is the center value in a distribution list. For example, the median of 1, 2, 3, 4, and 5 is 3 because 50% of the values lie before it and 50% after it in the distribution. The mode is the value that occurs most frequently in the data set. For example, the mode of 1, 1, 2, 3, 4, and 5 would be 1 because it is present more than any other number in the data set.

DEVELOPING A TOOL THAT COLLECTS STATISTICALLY VALID DATA

When developing a tool that collects statistically valid data, there are several steps to consider. To begin the process, it is imperative that management considers the resources to use in building the tool. Clinical enterprise data warehouses are an excellent place to start. These warehouses are typically governed by internal clinical informaticists, who have vetted the data and ensure that the data are valid for use. In many cases, the clinical enterprise data warehouses will also be governed by clinical advisory boards, who lend their input and approval of valid data sources. Once a valid clinical enterprise data warehouse or clinical repository is selected and it is determined that its data can be merged into a designed tool, then the development of that tool can commence. A SharePoint content repository is an excellent platform for tool development. SharePoint can be customized to meet the needs of a department as well as the needs of multiple departments. The SharePoint workflow process is a valuable asset when intradepartmental collaboration is a must. For example, a coding audit tool may be built in SharePoint, using its features of workflow between the audit department, the coding department, and the billing department.

RELATIONAL DATABASES

In healthcare, multiple different types of data are collected — financial data, administrative data, and clinical data. The data are collected and stored in databases, with relational databases being one of the most common types used in healthcare. Being knowledgeable of relational databases enhances collaborative efforts between health information management (HIM) and information technology (IT) professionals. Input from HIM professionals pertaining to work flow, data definitions, data quality, and health information privacy/confidentiality is needed, and input from IT pertaining to relational database organization is needed to enhance collaborative discussions. Relational databases are organized into relational tables, with rows and columns of recorded data. Each field in the table describes an attribute of a record, such as a patient's last name, first name, medical record number, date of birth, etc. One table is also known as a flat file. A relational database consists of two or more related tables that are linked to one another

60

through a unique identifier (e.g., medical record number). Through the linkage of multiple related tables, many results may be yielded that can enhance decision-making processes.

DATA MAPPING

Data mapping can be defined as the process of linking two distinct or disparate data sources for the purpose of exchanging data or information. It can be referenced as data sharing and/or interoperability. Data mapping requires frequent integrity checks or validation whether through continuous monitoring mechanisms or auditing processes. Accurate mapping should provide uniform, reliable, and complete data, which constitutes its integrity. Challenges of data mapping that can affect its integrity may be: drop-down pick lists, computer-assisted code assignments, templates that omit important fields, inaccurate workflows, failure to update maps, interface engines, etc. Validity testing in the production environment should be performed routinely to verify that the map is still meeting its intended purpose. Identification of inaccurate mapping results should be investigated for root cause(s) and should be resolved promptly.

MAPPING PATHWAYS

Through the use of a code map, one is able to either forward map or backward map. Forward mapping is when the ICD-9 code is available and an ICD-10 code is needed, and backward mapping is the opposite — an ICD-10 code is available, but an ICD-9 code is needed. It is important to understand that general equivalence mappings (GEMs) do not necessarily have a 1:1 match between the two code sets. For example, it is estimated that less than 25% of ICD-9 codes can be mapped to an ICD-10 code. Obviously, there are ICD-9 codes that map to multiple ICD-10 codes, and this is known as one-to-many mapping, and in these cases, the multiple ICD-10 codes are more specific than the ICD-9 codes. Because there is a GEM concept for one-to-many mapping, it is important to understand that there is a many-to-one mapping. In these cases, more than one ICD-9 code is required to provide a match to a single ICD-10 code.

METHODS TO ENSURE EFFECTIVE AUDIT REPORTS

An audit report is created to be read, followed by actions being implemented. An audit report is the communication tool that, with excellent writing skills, can be the catalyst to effectively enforce compliance. An effective audit report, however, should not begin at the end of an audit. Communication between the auditor and the auditee(s) should start with preaudit meetings, through which the audit process and scope are defined, and the auditee is given the opportunity to express their thoughts and concerns. Open communication should be held throughout the audit fieldwork, factoring pertinent information attained into the audit report. A draft audit report should be provided to the audited manager(s) prior to a closing face-to-face meeting, allowing the manager(s) time to prepare a response. The use of audit report templates can also help the auditor write an effective message. Templates promote timeliness and conciseness in report writing.

HEALTHCARE COMPLIANCE AUDIT REPORT COMPONENTS

A healthcare compliance audit report is the end product of an investigation into designated healthcare practices and its associated compliance risks. The structure of a healthcare compliance audit report should include the following components: background, scope, methodology, regulatory guidance, objectives, audit results, recommendations, and auditee response. The background covers the reason for the audit, such as identified errors, identified workflow process issues, regulatory focus, etc. The scope explains the population, the sample size, references, and time frame. The methodology addresses the steps of the investigation (i.e., interviews, resources reviewed, data analytics, etc.). Regulatory guidance provides the foundation for the audit's objectives (i.e., Medicare's national coverage determinations/local coverage determinations, Office of Inspector General Annual Audit Plan, etc.). Audit results focus on noncompliant issues described as error percentages and workflow inefficiencies, and recommendations are provided to help guide auditees in the development of their response.

Revenue Cycle Management

HEALTH RECORD IDENTIFICATION SYSTEMS

For paper or electronic health records, each record must have a unique identifier of either an alphabetical or numerical source. The unique health record number is assigned at the time of hospital admission or physician practice encounter and is used throughout the patient's treatment period at the corresponding facility. The simplest form of health record identification is alphabetical (primarily using the patient's name) and does not require cross-referencing to a master patient index (MPI) numerical identifier. Patient confidentiality is a concern for an alphabetical system, and as such, is not highly used or encouraged. A numerical numbering system is encouraged because patient privacy is better protected. The numerical numbering system does require cross referencing to an MPI. There are two types of numbering systems: serial and unit. Serial numbering uses a new number for each patient visit, and it is not widely used. Unit numbering uses the same number repeatedly throughout the entire patient visit, and is advantageous in that it distinguishes each patient from all other patients, promotes centralization of record documentation, and provides the clinical staff with a complete picture of the patient's health history.

CREATION OF HEALTH RECORD NUMBERS

Health record numbers may be created according to various schematics. One option is to assign sequential numbers. Sequential numbers are numbers that are assigned in a chronological sequence. For example, if patient A receives a number assignment of 56892, then patient B would receive a number assignment of 56893. Alphanumeric numbering is a combination of letters and numbers. This numbering schematic should only be used for small healthcare entities because it does not offer numerous options. The alphabet only has 26 letters, and there are only 10 numerical figures including 0 through 9. Relational numbering offers a number that is significant to each patient because it can use a birth date, gender codes, and geographic codes, among others. Social Security numbering is another numbering schematic that is not highly recommended, primarily due to privacy concerns, identity theft concerns, and the fact that some individuals residing in the United States do not have a Social Security number.

TERMINAL DIGIT FILING

The most popular paper health record filing system used is terminal digit filing. In terminal digit, six to seven digits will be assigned and divided into three sections. The terminal digit number is read backwards, from right to left, two digits at a time. In other words, the primary digits are the first two digits on the right-hand side. The secondary digits are the next two digits in the middle, and the tertiary digits are the final two digits on the left-hand side. When filing a paper health record, the clerk will search for the primary section within 100 primary sections. For example, if the record number is 24-28-50, then the clerk will initially locate section 50. Within each primary section are 100 secondary sections. Using the same number above,

63

once section 50 is located, then the clerk would locate section 28. Finally, within the 28-50 section, the clerk would file the record in numerical order according to the tertiary number. In this example, 24 would require the record to be filed between 23 and 25.

INVOLVEMENT OF HIM PROFESSIONALS IN THE REVENUE CYCLE

A standard health information management (HIM) function in terms of revenue cycle involvement is the coding manager's responsibility to monitor the DNFB. DNFB is the acronym for discharged, not final billed. DNFB is not the same as accounts receivable (A/R). The difference between the two functions is that accounts in DNFB status are unbilled (even though the patient has been discharged from the hospital), whereas accounts that are pending in A/R are billed but the monies have not been received, denied, or settled yet. Another way to understand this concept is: If it's due to be received, it's a receivable, and it can't be due if it hasn't been billed. The number of days that accounts are pending in A/R is a measure monitored by patient financial services. The number of days that accounts are pending in DNFB status or days in revenue outstanding is a measure monitored by HIM. There are certain components of DNFB and A/R that must be monitored consistently. For example, HIM must monitor the discharge date to code date, looking for reasons why coding has not been completed (e.g., unavailable records, missing documentation, etc.). For A/R, patient financial services must monitor the bill date to collection date, the primary pay date to the secondary payer's pay date, self-pay portions, and posting payments.

WAYS HIM WORKFLOW PROCESSES MAY IMPEDE THE REVENUE CYCLE

Health information management (HIM) workflow processes can impede the revenue cycle. These HIM workflow processes should be assessed and monitored for inefficiencies. For example, the following list contains areas to be managed closely by HIM professionals: timeliness of record receipt, monitoring of the unbilled list of records, assessment of the unbilled list for duplicative records, evaluation of inefficient communication methods with patient financial services regarding delays, assessment of coding productivity standards and coding accuracy standards, and assessment of the reasons for missing documentation needed to complete coding.

ICD-10-PCS FORMAT

ICD-10-PCS is formatted in three sections: tables, index, and list of codes. The index is an alphabetic listing of procedures/operations. Codes are organized in the index according to the general type of procedure. Of note, the index only provides the first 3 to 4 characters of a procedural code. The remaining characters are located in the tables, and thus the tables must be referenced in order to assign a valid 7-digit code. The tables are designed in rows that provide options for characters 4 through 7 in the development of valid code combinations. The list of codes is a comprehensive list of all procedural codes along with their descriptions. The process of assigning an ICD-10-PCS code begins with the coder accessing the index in order to locate the appropriate table, and then referencing that table to locate the remaining characters for code completion.

64

CODING GUIDELINE CHANGES BETWEEN THE ICD-9 AND ICD-10 SYSTEMS

For the majority of the official coding guidance available to coders, the guidance remained the same with the transition from ICD-9 to ICD-10. There were a few significant changes, however, and coders should be informed of these changes to ensure compliant coding. A few of these changes are as follows:

- Neoplasm-related anemia: In ICD-9, anemia was sequenced as the principal diagnosis, followed by the malignancy code(s). In ICD-10, official coding guidance now states to sequence the malignancy as the principal diagnosis. Depending upon the type of malignancy, the financial impact of this coding guidance change can either be a negative or a positive impact.
- Hemiplegia/Hemiparesis: In ICD-9, unilateral weakness could not be coded as hemiparesis with a stroke (unless confirmed through a query). In ICD-10, unilateral weakness with a stroke is assumed to be hemiparesis/hemiplegia.
- Coronary artery disease (CAD): In ICD-9, unspecified CAD in a patient with a past surgical history of coronary artery bypass grafting would be coded to an unspecified coronary artery. In ICD-10, the default for the unspecified component goes to a native artery.

ROOT OPERATIONS WITH OBJECTIVE TO PULL OUT/OFF ALL OR PORTION OF A BODY PART

There are five root operations in ICD-10-PCS that remove some or all of a body part. All five are done with no replacement of the body part or tissue. The five root operations are listed as follows (with their differences in bold):

Root Operation	Purpose of the Procedure	Site of Procedure
Excision	Cut out or off	Portion of a body part
Resection	Cut out or off	Entire body part
Detachment	Cut out or off	Extremities only; exclusive to amputations
Destruction	Eradicate/Destroy	Body part is not removed; rather, it is destroyed
Extraction	Pull out with force	Portion of a body part or entire body part

Of note, there are 31 root operations in total, divided into 9 groups that are similar. The remaining eight groups are procedures that (1) remove solids/fluids/gases, (2) cut or separate only, (3) put in or put back some or all of a body part, (4) alter the diameter of a tubular structure, (5) include a device, (6) involve examination only, (7) include other repairs, and (8) include other objectives.

ROOT OPERATIONS INVOLVING A DEVICE

There are six root operations in ICD-10-PCS that always involve a device. For the purposes of ICD-10-PCS coding, a device is defined as an appliance or material that remains in the body or on the body after the procedure. The six root operations are listed as follows (with their differences in bold):

Root Operation	Purpose of the Procedure	Example

65

Insertion	Addition of a nonbiological device	Foley catheter placement
Replacement	Addition of a device that replaces a body part	Phacoemulsification with an intraocular lens (IOL) implant
Supplement	Addition of a device that reinforces a body part	Umbilical hernia repair with mesh
Change	Exchange of a device	Tracheostomy tube exchange
Removal	Take out a device	Removal of endotracheal tube
Revision	Modification of a malfunctioning device	Adjustment of a pacemaker lead

UPPER AND LOWER BODY PARTS IN ICD-10-PCS CODING

In ICD-10-PCS coding, in some scenarios, a coder will encounter documentation referring to "upper" or "lower" body parts. For example, the documentation may refer to upper or lower arteries or veins. When the terms "upper" or "lower" are used in reference to body parts, the dividing anatomical line between the two body locations is the diaphragm. Understanding this general guideline will aid the coder in selecting the correct body system that represents character #2 of the procedural code.

PROPERLY SEQUENCING ICD-10-CM CODES FOR INPATIENTS

The sequencing of diagnostic codes is key to accurate diagnosis-related group (DRG) assignment. Code sequencing drives the selection of the principal diagnosis, which is the most important code assignment a coder will make. Of course, the principal diagnosis must be selected at the highest level of specificity, followed by secondary diagnoses. Some secondary diagnoses are classified as complications/comorbidities or major complications/comorbidities. They, too, will impact the DRG assignment. The relationship between the principal and secondary diagnoses is factored into DRG grouper logic. Coders must be vigilant in reviewing all healthcare documentation in order to select and sequence all diagnoses correctly for the most compliant and financially impactful order. Of note, it is possible for an ICD-10-PCS procedure code to impact the DRG assignment.

PURPOSE OF RESEQUENCING CODES IN ICD-10

The American Health Information Management Association has an established Standards of Ethical Coding that coders are expected to follow. The standards emphasize that all healthcare data elements (e.g., diagnosis codes, procedure codes, etc.) must be reported completely and accurately and supported by healthcare documentation. One standard points out that coders are not to change codes for the purpose of inappropriately increasing payment. Therefore, it is important that coders apply official coding guidelines correctly and only resequence the order of codes according to ICD-10 rules. Resequencing codes can either have a positive or negative financial impact because the diagnosis-related group (DRG) selection can change to a higher or lower paying rate. If documentation does not support the DRG change, the healthcare organization could be accused of upcoding for financial gain. This can place the healthcare organization at risk of being found guilty of fraudulent claim billing.

APPROPRIATE OCCASIONS TO RESEQUENCE ICD-10-CM CODES FOR OPTIMAL REIMBURSEMENT

When assigning ICD-10-CM codes for an inpatient encounter, there are occasions wherein it would be appropriate to resequence the codes in order to obtain optimal reimbursement. This usually occurs when referencing the ICD-10-CM Official Guidelines for Coding and Reporting for selection of the principal diagnosis (Section IIC). The Section IIC guideline is used when two or more diagnoses equally meet the definition for the principal diagnosis. Of course, the coder must ensure that both diagnoses were determined to be the cause of the admission and both were treated therapeutically or "worked up" with diagnostic procedures. If all of these factors are met, then either diagnosis may be sequenced first. An example of when this guideline could be applied follows: A patient was admitted with exacerbation of chronic obstructive pulmonary disease and acute on chronic diastolic heart failure. Both conditions were treated with intravenous meds, oxygen therapy, and respiratory therapy. Because both diagnoses were the reason for the patient's admission and both were treated equally, either one could be selected as the principal diagnosis. Subsequently, the one associated with a higher-weighted diagnosis-related group should be chosen as the principal diagnosis.

POA INDICATOR

Present on admission (POA) indicators are a reporting requirement for healthcare providers. The Deficit Reduction Act of 2005 mandated that providers report whether diseases were present on admission or not. The intent of the indicators is to differentiate between conditions that are present at the time of admission and those that develop during the inpatient admission. Financial incentives are available for providers who reduce the number of hospital-acquired conditions (not present on admission). There are five indicators to select from: "Y" = yes, POA; "N" = no, not POA; "U" = unknown, documentation is insufficient to make a determination; "W" = clinically undetermined; and "1" = exempt from POA reporting. In the instance where a combination code identifies both a chronic condition as well as its acute exacerbation, the following best practice should be followed: Assign "N" if any part of the combination code was not POA; assign "Y" if all parts of the combination code were POA.

APR-DRGs AND MS-DRGs

APR-DRG is the acronym for all patient refined diagnosis-related groups, and MS-DRG is the acronym for Medicare severity diagnosis-related group. The major differences between APR-DRGs and MS-DRGs are as follows: severity classification structure, level of complexity, and clinical logic used. APR-DRGs factor in clinical logic in the form of severity of illness (SOI) and risk of mortality (ROM) measures. SOI measures describe the extent of an organ's loss of function, and ROM measures indicate the likelihood of patient death. There are diagnoses that impact reimbursement in the APR system but do not impact reimbursement in the DRG system. For example, in the APR system, portal hypertension is considered to be a moderate severity of illness measure, but in the DRG system, it is not considered to be a complication/comorbidity and does not impact reimbursement.

HACs

A hospital-acquired condition (HAC) is an unfavorable condition (e.g., an infection, development of a decubitus ulcer, etc.) that occurs during the hospitalization and adversely affects the patient's health and course of treatment. Another way to understand HACs is to think of them as complications or nosocomial infections/conditions. The Deficit Reduction Act of 2005 requires the reporting of conditions that are of a high cost or high volume and that could have potentially been prevented by following guidance from evidence-based outcomes. A current list of HACs is maintained by the Centers for Medicare & Medicaid Services (CMS) and can be accessed through CMS.gov. The ultimate goal in identifying HACs is to provide an incentive to hospitals to reduce HACs. CMS has instituted the Hospital-Acquired Condition Reduction Program (HACRP). HACRP adjust payments to healthcare entities that rank in the worst performing quartile of all hospitals. Nationwide, hospitals can be compared online through the Medicare.gov Hospital Compare page.

HACRP

The Hospital-Acquired Condition Reduction Program (HACRP) is mandated by the Affordable Care Act (effective October 1, 2014). The Centers for Medicare and Medicaid Services calculates HAC scores for all inpatient prospective payment system hospitals. The scoring is a ratio of the number of HACS to the number of eligible patients based upon certain quality measures. The measures include pressure ulcers, pneumothorax, catheter-related bloodstream infections, and post-op hip fractures, to name a few. A HAC is determined through the application of a present on admission (POA) indicator. If a diagnosis is POA, then it would not be considered to be acquired in the hospital. However, if a diagnosis is not POA, then it would be considered to be hospital acquired. For example, if a patient develops a pulmonary embolism after a surgery, the POA indicator for the pulmonary embolism would be "no," and this would fall under the pulmonary embolism HAC. For some HACs, the hospital will not receive financial reimbursement; this is a type of incentive to encourage hospitals to prevent or control the number of HACs.

ABNs

ABN is the acronym for advanced beneficiary notice of noncoverage (Form CMS-R-131). An ABN is provided to a patient when the healthcare entity determines that a planned procedure is not medically necessary and therefore will not be covered for reimbursement purposes. An ABN must be provided to the patient in advance of a planned procedure or service in order to give the patient time to consider his/her options and then to make a decision on how best to proceed. In order to determine if a procedure or service is medically necessary (and thus covered by Medicare), healthcare representatives should access either the Medicare Coverage Database or local/national coverage determinations. The ABN gives patients the options to choose to proceed with the procedure/service and accept financial responsibility or to disagree to follow through with the procedure/service. Appeal options to Medicare are available as well.

CHARGE CAPTURE AUDIT

Charge capture is a revenue-producing function in which clinical departments enter charges for services provided. The charges may be generated by selecting specific charges from a department-specific list or from clinical documentation or from an order initiated by the physician. The charges may be automatically "hard coded" to a patient's account, or they may be manually entered. Charges entered by the clinical staff must be audited for accuracy, especially when considering potential penalties associated with the False Claims Act for noncompliance. The primary objective of a charge capture audit is to confirm the compliance with documentation, accuracy of Current Procedural Terminology (CPT) codes associated with charges, accuracy of service units billed, and accuracy of the fair market value of charges. Some of the risks associated with a charge capture audit may include the following:

- Charge entry on the wrong encounter.
- Insufficient documentation to support the charge(s).
- Inaccurate charge capture.
- Missed charge(s). Interface issues resulting in missed charges.
- Incorrect CPT codes associated with charges.

PDX

The principal diagnosis (PDX) is one of the most important code assignments a coder can select. In many instances, the PDX will be the "driver" behind the diagnosis-related group (DRG) (also known as "disease groupings") selection. Of course, the secondary diagnosis (SDX), which may be designated as a major complication or comorbidity or a complication/comorbidity, can impact the DRG assignment. Regardless of which diagnosis (or sometimes even procedure) code is the "driver" behind the DRG assignment, the PDX is still of upmost importance for correct selection. The PDX is defined by the Uniform Hospital Discharge Data Set as the condition established after study to be responsible for causing the patient's admission to the hospital. There are many coding guidelines to consider when determining the PDX, and its assignment can be a source of disagreement between coders and auditors (internal and/or external). Therefore, it is essential that a coder reviews the entire medical record for the complete picture of the patient's case and determine, after study, what caused the patient's admission.

CHARACTERS FOR MEDICAL AND SURGICAL PROCEDURES

Medical and surgical procedural codes are composed of 7 characters. The characters and their meanings follow. The first character represents 4 different *sections*: 0, med/surg; 1, obstetrics; 2, placement; and 3, administration. (The majority of procedural codes are categorized in the med/surg section.) The second character represents the *body system* (e.g., cardiology, respiratory). The third character represents the *root operation*, also known as the objective of the procedure. The fourth character represents the *body part* where the procedure is performed (e.g., stomach, brain). The fifth character represents the *approach* or method to reach the procedure site (e.g., open, percutaneous). The sixth character represents the *device* used during the procedure (e.g., implant). The seventh character represents the *qualifier* that provides additional information about the procedure.

The following mnemonic can help you to memorize the seven characters:

Section	Sam
Body System	Baked
Root Operation	Raspberry
Body Part	Bagels
Approach	And
Device	Dandelion
Qualifier	Quiche

SEPSIS

Sepsis is known to be one of the most challenging conditions to code. Sepsis is a complex condition with multiple terms (sepsis, systemic inflammatory response syndrome [SIRS], severe sepsis, and septic shock), which can confuse coding applications. The following are tips on how to alleviate the confusion and code sepsis accurately:

- To code sepsis, two codes are required: one for the underlying infection and one for the sepsis or severe sepsis.
- When acute organ dysfunction occurs with sepsis (e.g., acute respiratory failure, acute renal failure, acute liver failure, etc.), either code R65.20 (severe sepsis without septic shock) or R65.21 (severe sepsis with septic shock) must also be coded.
- It is important to remember to follow the tabular instructions to code "first" the underlying infection (e.g., urinary tract infection, pneumonia, etc.), when applicable.
- Coding of sepsis in a newborn is different because only one code is assigned — 771.81.
- If the organism causing the sepsis (e.g., *Streptococcus*) is known, it should be coded also.

FRACTURES

Coding of fractures requires careful review of documentation for multiple details. To begin, identification of whether fractures are pathological or traumatic in origin must be noted. Fractures must be identified as either open or closed and displaced or nondisplaced. Fracture codes will also include reference to anatomical site, laterality (e.g., right or left), routine or delayed healing, nonunion or malunion, and type of encounter (e.g., initial, subsequent, or sequela). Each of these aspects will impact the various seventh characters of a fracture code; for example, an initial

70

encounter for a closed fracture will result in a seventh character of "A," but an initial encounter for an open fracture will result in a seventh character of "B."

VENTILATOR TIME

The following are tips on how to code continuous ventilator time management accurately: Assign a procedural code for ventilator time based upon "hours" and not "days." Search the clinical documentation thoroughly for the intubation time and the extubation time. These times may be documented by the emergency department physician, attending physician, or intubating physician in the emergency department record, the history and physical, or progress notes. A respiratory therapist or nursing staff may document the times in a computerized abstracting system (e.g., Meditech). When the intubation and extubation times are identified, calculations should be performed to determine if the ventilation time exceeded 96 hours. For example, if documentation supports that endotracheal intubation occurred on February 2 at 09:50 and extubation occurred on February 6 at 11:53, then the patient was on the ventilator for 98 hours. It is important to know that the ventilator-weaning period (when the patient is being withdrawn from the ventilator) is also included in the continuous ventilator time.

TRANSBRONCHIAL LUNG BIOPSIES

Bronchoscopies with transbronchial lung biopsies can be rather tricky to code. The following are tips on how to code transbronchial lung biopsies accurately:

- If a biopsy is performed of a lesion seen via the bronchoscope, then most likely the lesion is NOT in the lung.
- If fluoroscopy is used as part of the bronchoscopy to visualize the lesion, then the lesion probably is in the lung.
- If the documentation states that there is an infiltrate or lung lesion being biopsied, it probably is in the lung.
- If mediastinal or hilar lymph nodes are being biopsied, it probably is NOT in the lung.
- If the patient develops a pneumothorax after the procedure, then the lesion was probably in the lung.
- If a pathology report does not state alveolar or lung tissue, this does NOT necessarily exclude the possibility of a lung biopsy because poor tissue sampling may have occurred from an actual lung biopsy.

PHYSICIAN QUERIES

INTENT

A physician query is a tool of communication between clinical documentation information specialists/coders and physicians to clarify incomplete, ambiguous, or conflicting documentation in the medical record. The intention of the communication tool is to facilitate completeness, accuracy, consistency, and timely documentation for coding and reporting practices. Queries are an essential tool that provides additional clarification that allows coding and reporting to the highest level of specificity. It is best for the physician's query to be maintained as a permanent part of the medical record because it is considered to be supporting documentation for assigned codes.

INITIATION

There are several reasons why a coder would initiate a physician's query. If a diagnosis and/or procedure has been determined to meet the American Hospital Association's ICD-10 Official Guidelines for Coding and Reporting, but the diagnosis and/or procedure has not been clearly stated within the documentation, then a query may be necessary. The reasons why initiation of a query may occur would be either of the following: (1) when a present on admission (POA) indicator is not clearly stated and the coder must know this information in order to meet the federal requirement to report POA status or (2) when conflicting, ambiguous, or incomplete documentation is present. Query templates may be a helpful tool for coders to use when initiating queries because they promote query standardization.

Issues such as legibility, completeness, clarity, or consistency may be what prompts the initiation of a query. The query may be done either concurrently by a clinical documentation information (CDI) specialist or retrospectively by a coder. Physician queries must be phrased in such a way that it does not appear that the CDI specialist or coder is leading the physician to a certain diagnosis. Physician queries must provide clinical indicators from the existing documentation that explains the CDI specialist's or coder's reasoning to the queried physician.

REQUIRED COMPONENTS

A physician query should include certain components in order to be a valid and/or compliant query. These components include the following:

- Name of the contact individual submitting the query.
- Patient's date of service.
- Patient's name.
- Medical record number.
- Account number.
- Date of the query.
- Name of the physician being queried.
- Clinical indicators pertinent to the condition/diagnosis/procedure in question.
- Statement of the issue in the form of a question.

Examples of when queries may be issued are as follows:

- Determine if a diagnosis was present on admission.
- Clarify what specific organism was the cause and effect of an infectious disease.
- Clarify the severity of asthma.
- Clarify the particular stage of chronic kidney disease.
- Clarify if a diagnosis was ruled in or ruled out.

72

- Determine which diagnosis or procedure is applicable when conflicting information exists.
- Clarify whether or not pneumonia was caused by aspiration.

STANDARDIZED FORMS

The use of standardized physician query forms by coders and/or clinical documentation improvement specialists is an efficient way to obtain compliant queries. Standardized queries should be created based upon disease processes or circumstances that are most likely to require a query (e.g., sepsis, acuity of respiratory failure, specificity of renal failure, whether a diagnosis was ruled in or ruled out, etc.). Through the use of standardized forms with specified clinical indicators, three objectives should be accomplished: (1) overall documentation improvement should be noted, (2) potential coding errors due to poor documentation practices should be avoided, and (3) potential compliance issues related to leading queries should be mitigated.

FORMATTING OPTIONS

There are several ways to generate a query. Compliant query forms will allow for open-ended questions, multiple-choice query formats, and/or limited yes/no query formats. An example of an open-ended query might appear in this format: "Based upon your clinical judgment, please provide a diagnosis that represents the following clinical indicators: temperature, 102°; cellulitis around ankle with open wound; white blood cell (WBC) count, 15,000." An example of a multiple-choice query might appear in this format: "Per the Discharge Summary, the patient has congestive heart failure (CHF). Can the CHF be further specified as one of the following: (1) acute systolic CHF, (2) acute on chronic systolic CHF, (3) acute diastolic CHF, (4) acute on chronic diastolic CHF, or (5) undetermined?" An example of a yes/no query might appear in this format: "Was the sepsis documented in the discharge summary present on admission? Yes, no, clinically unable to determine."

POLICIES

Physician queries are an integral part of clinical documentation improvement programs in healthcare institutions today. In order to standardize methods for physician query processes, query policies are recommended. Effective policies should establish query guidelines pertaining to the four "W's": (1) who (e.g., which physician is responsible for providing clarity?), (2) what (e.g., which diagnosis or procedure is unclear?), (3) when (e.g., when is a query needed?), and (4) why (e.g., is documentation unclear or conflicting?). Policies should address any compliance-related issues (e.g., avoidance of leading a physician to the selection of a desired diagnosis). Query policies should explain appropriate means of following up on unanswered queries (e.g., time frames, acceptable number of queries to issue, etc.).

CLINICAL INDICATORS

Compliant coding is dependent upon the accuracy and completeness of documentation. In some cases, healthcare documentation is not sufficient to support code assignments, and in those cases, physician queries are necessary. Queries must contain certain elements, and clinical indicators are one of the elements. Clinical indicators refer to clinical clues, such as elevated temperature, abnormal vital signs, elevated white blood count levels, etc., that could indicate or support certain diagnoses. For example, if a provider fails to document the diagnosis of sepsis, but there are clinical indicators that point to its diagnosis, a query might be warranted. The coder or clinical documentation improvement specialist might include the following clinical indicators in the query: temperature, 103°; white blood cell count, 18,500; blood pressure, 70/40 (hypotension). These three clinical clues might indicate the diagnosis of sepsis, and the physician would consider these indicators to make a decision.

PROCESS TO FOLLOW WHEN CONFLICTING DOCUMENTATION EXISTS

Some patients admitted to an inpatient status in the hospital will be assessed by multiple physicians. Inevitably, the documentation of the various physicians will conflict. For example, the attending physician may document acute renal "failure," but the nephrology consultant documents acute renal "disease." Because failure and disease in this particular case equate to different codes, the coder will need clarification, and that clarification is best achieved through the initiation of a query. The query would need to reveal the conflicting information and ask for the final decision as to which diagnosis is correct. Other clinical indicators should be a part of the query in order to demonstrate to the physician why the information is conflicting. For example, in this acute renal failure versus disease scenario, the coder may choose to include the clinical indicators pertaining to a rise in the blood urea nitrogen/creatinine as well as the urine output amounts.

CLINICAL CRITERIA TO INCLUDE IN QUERIES TO IDENTIFY CONDITIONS OR DISEASES
ACUTE KIDNEY FAILURE

When issuing a physician query, a coder or clinical documentation improvement specialist should include clinical indicators for the physician's consideration when trying to determine if a condition or disease process is present. In the case of acute kidney failure (or acute kidney injury), the following clinical indicators could be used: creatinine value > or = 0.3 mg/dl increase within 48 hours. Creatinine value > or = 1.5× increase from baseline. Urine output <0.5 ml/kg/hr for > or = 6 hours. It is possible for acute kidney failure/injury to be further specified as acute tubular necrosis (ATN), renal cortical necrosis (RCN), or renal papillary necrosis (RPN). With further specificity, the diagnosis-related group (DRG) could potentially change with an increase in the reimbursement amount. To help in deciding if one of these more specific diagnoses is applicable, the physician could be queried as follows: For ATN, use the clinical indicator(s) of hypotension, sepsis, or toxic ingestion, if present. For RCN, use the clinical indicator(s) of sepsis, rejection of a transplanted kidney, poisoning, or pancreatitis, if present. For RPN, use the clinical indicator(s) of diabetic nephropathy, kidney infection, rejection of a kidney transplant, or sickle cell anemia, if present.

CHF

When issuing a physician query, a coder or clinical documentation improvement (CDI) specialist should include clinical indicators for the physician's consideration when trying to determine if a condition or disease process is present. In the case of congestive heart failure (CHF), if the physician has documented that the patient has CHF, then the following clinical indicators could be used to determine further specificity pertaining to the type of CHF and/or the acuity of the CHF:

- Increase in respiratory rate.
- Evidence of pleural effusion on chest X-ray.
- Clinical symptoms of swelling in the lower extremities, increased work of breathing, or shortness of breath.

The aim of the query is threefold: (1) Determine if the CHF is systolic, diastolic, or combined systolic/diastolic, (2) determine if the CHF is acute, chronic, or acute on chronic, and (3) determine if the CHF is due to hypertension, rheumatic fever, or a specific valvular disease.

ACUTE RESPIRATORY FAILURE

When issuing a physician query, a coder or clinical documentation improvement specialist should include clinical indicators for the physician's consideration when trying to determine if a condition or disease process is present. In the case of acute respiratory failure, the following clinical indicators could be used in the query:

- Respiratory rate > 35/min.
- Hypoxia or hypercapnia.
- Cyanosis.
- Diffuse bilateral pulmonary infiltrates.
- Additional oxygen requirements.
- Additional respiratory therapy.
- Invasive or noninvasive mechanical ventilation.
- Increased work of breathing. For patients with previously normal lungs, a PO_2 value <55 mmHG, a PCO_2 value >50 mmHg.
- For patients with previously abnormal lungs, a pH value <7.35 with a PCO_2 value >50 mmHg.

To determine if chronic respiratory failure is a valid diagnosis, the patient should have been on oxygen for 24 hours/day or have been on a chronic ventilator. There may be evidence of cor pulmonale. There may be evidence of chronically elevated bicarbonate levels.

LEADING QUERY

A leading query can be defined as one that is not supported by the clinical elements contained within the medical record, or it can be defined as a query that directs a healthcare provider to a specific diagnosis or procedure. By leading a provider to a specific diagnosis or procedure is an unbalanced approach because it appears to prompt the provider to make only one decision. A coder or clinical documentation improvement (CDI) specialist should never suggest only one diagnostic or procedural option because coders/CDI specialists are not credentialed healthcare providers.

EXAMPLES

Leading provider/physician queries are not acceptable in healthcare. The following are examples of inappropriate leading queries:

- A query that provides the physician with options that only lead to additional reimbursement.
- A query that does not contain all the required clinical indicators, which give the full clinical details of the patient's condition.
- A query wherein the statements are directive in nature, such as indicating what the provider should document, rather than querying the provider for his/her professional determination of the clinical facts.
- A query that leads the provider to one desired outcome.
- A query that omits reasonable clinically supported options.
- A query that omits an option that no additional documentation or clarification may be provided.

CDI TIPS LIBRARY

With the implementation of the ICD-10 coding classification system, the expectation for more in-depth documentation became a reality. The role of clinical documentation improvement (CDI) specialists has expanded as a result. The CDI specialist must be able to identify the level of documentation specificity needed with ICD-10 coding applications. Management of the CDI process should include the creation of a CDI tips library. Once documentation improvement areas are identified, they should be added to the CDI tips library for reference sources as well as for training purposes. The process of developing a CDI tips library should include going through each chapter of both the ICD-10-CM and ICD-10-PCS manuals for the purpose of identifying diagnoses, conditions, and procedures in need of specific documentation. For example, the diagnosis of congestive heart failure (CHF) should be added to the library along with documentation tips to support the type of CHF and its acuity level. The documentation tips for CHF may include any of the following: (1) document whether the CHF is of systolic or diastolic origin, (2) document if the CHF is acute, chronic, or acute on chronic, and/or (3) document any associated diagnoses.

CONTRIBUTIONS OF CASE MANAGERS TO IMPROVED HOSPITAL PERFORMANCE

Hospital case managers are key employees when it comes to ensuring that every patient receives appropriate care and that hospitals receive reimbursement for services rendered. Case managers make significant contributions to the hospital's overall performance. They may do so through the following methods: improved patient outcomes, reduced readmissions, and enhancement of claims management. The primary responsibility of a case manager is to improve patient outcomes.

Effective follow-up through scheduled appointments in the outpatient setting can help to ensure improved patient outcomes, and medication management after hospitalization can promote improved patient outcomes. These efforts can reduce readmission rates of patients to inpatient acute care. A vital part of the case manager's role is to ensure that each patient's stay is medically necessary, which in turn reduces the risks of claim denials. If a patient's stay is determined by Medicare as being medically unnecessary, the hospital loses a large sum of money. Hence, it is obvious that the case manager is instrumental in reducing denials on the back end by ensuring the medical necessity on the front end.

APPEALS PROCESS FOR DENIED CLAIM

Before a denied healthcare claim is appealed, there are several steps the healthcare entity should take. The steps include the following:

1. Reviewing all available documentation for completeness.
2. Reviewing the content of the documentation for accuracy and/or inconsistencies and determining if further information is needed through queries, updates, or additional documentation.
3. Include supporting documentation from providers of care to provide clarification.
4. Review regulatory guidance related to the denial for the purpose of using the information in the appeal letter.

Once these preliminary steps are completed, the process shifts to composing the appeal. The appeal letter should include supporting clinical documentation. Any necessary forms required for the appeal should be completed and included with submission of the appeal letter. Time frames for submission should be closely followed to avoid missing the deadline. In the appeal letter, point out specific key information that is crucial to reversing the denial (e.g., medication administration, ancillary test results, key provider terminology in support of code assignments, etc.). A well-written and documentation-supported appeal letter should reverse the denial.

IDEAL COMPOSITION OF A DENIAL MANAGEMENT TEAM

Denial management is a static function of a healthcare entity. Denials are not caused by bad debt, charitable care, or contractual adjustments. Rather, denials are the fault of the healthcare provider. In other words, when a claim is denied, it is because the healthcare entity was not compliant with billing practices. To keep the volume of denials under control, a denial management team must be involved in the revenue cycle process. The team should be comprised of representatives from the following departments: patient financial services, health information management, registration/scheduling, case management, compliance, charge services, information technology, and decision support. The team's objectives should be to determine common reasons for denials, contributions to denials, and tracking and trending of denials. Common reasons for denials may include submission of claims to the wrong payer or wrong address, coordination of benefits, ineligibility,

77

duplicate claims, and medical necessity issues. Contributions to denials may be attributed to inexperienced staff, registration errors, eligibility issues, benefit reductions, lack of precertification, and coding errors. To track and trend denials, a spreadsheet or log containing the following information should be maintained: denial reason, payer's name, account number, denied charges, date of denial resolution, date of claim resubmission, and end result.

HIM REPRESENTATIVES' SPECIFIC ROLE IN DENIALS MANAGEMENT PROCESS

Health information management (HIM) representatives must be involved in the denials management process. Denials management is not a function that is only addressed by the revenue cycle department. It is a collaborative multidisciplinary process aimed at determining common reasons for denials, contributions to denials, and tracking and trending of denials. HIM representatives' specific role should focus upon the following responsibilities:

- Assist in edit rejections prior to dropping the final claim. These edits may be outpatient code editor or National Correct Coding Initiative edits that alert coders to potential billing issues during the coding process.
- Issue physician queries before billing when coding is not supported by the existing documentation.
- Identify charge description master (CDM) errors in association with code assignments. These may be identified when documentation supports the code assignment for a type of procedure but the charges for that procedure were not assigned in the CDM and therefore were missing from the claim.
- Contribute to the appeal process for denials that are not substantiated by providing documentation to prove the denial is invalid.
- Distribute new compliance rules published by external agencies pertaining to coding and/or billing processes. The purpose of this responsibility is to provide the revenue cycle team with current education and training.

AVOIDING MEDICAL NECESSITY DENIALS

Medical necessity denials are commonly seen in healthcare facilities. The following are tips on how to prevent medical necessity denials:

- Establish policies for the departments involved (i.e., registration, health information management [HIM], patient financial services, etc.).
- Establish the expectation for providers to write an admission order 24 to 48 hours prior to a scheduled test or procedure.
- Require physicians to attach an advanced beneficiary notice (ABN) to an order, when applicable.
- Provide medical necessity education to physicians and responsible staff.
- Make available national coverage determinations and local coverage determinations to registration, HIM, and coding staff.
- Purchase and implement effective registration/ABN software.

MONITORING MEDICAL NECESSITY DATA

A medical necessity, evidence-based, clinical decision support system, such as InterQual, is a product used by healthcare entities nationwide. One objective of such a tool is to ensure the medical necessity of healthcare services. When denials related to the medical necessity of services are received from the payer, the case must be investigated by the healthcare entity. The first course of action would be to review the InterQual documentation and data collected for that stay in addition to reviewing medical record documentation. Through the use of these two sources, a valid appeal to the denial should be easy to compose. Additionally, monitoring medical necessity data can help to trend denial patterns and forecast future denial percentages, which then can aid management in the development of plans to reduce denials moving forward.

SI AND IS CRITERIA USED WHEN EVALUATING MEDICAL NECESSITY

Acute care inpatient and observation services for Medicare patients will be reviewed for medical necessity based upon severity of illness (SI) and intensity of service (IS) criteria. Criteria are specific for all body systems and for all care units (e.g., intensive care, medical beds, monitored beds, etc.). SI criteria will address the reasons for the patient's admission, if the patient's condition necessitates acute care, and if the patient has failed outpatient care. IS criteria will address what is being done for the patient in the acute care setting, and it will question if the treatment could be rendered at an alternate level of care (e.g., skilled nursing facility, rehabilitation services, home health care, etc.). Documentation in the electronic health record is critical to the support of acute inpatient care and in meeting SI/IS criteria. To extend a patient's stay in the inpatient acute care setting, documentation must support that the condition can only be treated as an inpatient and that the treatment is being provided for the acute condition.

AUDITING CODE ASSIGNMENTS

Healthcare entities should never assume that computer-assisted coding systems are 100% accurate. Therefore, it is imperative to implement a coding compliance program in which auditors review accounts on a daily basis. The volume of coded charts will far outweigh the number of auditors available to review; therefore, appropriate data analysis and filtering methods should be implemented to identify high-risk accounts. Once automated auditing tools identify the high-risk accounts, a systematic approach of auditing for compliant coding practices should occur. Any coding discrepancies should be conveyed to the coder for corrections and/or further discussion. After recommended corrections are made, rebills of corrected claims to the appropriate payer should occur.

EFFECTIVE CODING AUDIT PROGRAM

Effective coding compliance audit programs should incorporate the following elements, at a minimum: high-risk cases (e.g., excisional debridement, mechanical ventilation), cases with a diagnosis-related group (DRG) shift between ICD-9 and ICD-10 coding conventions, surgical procedure cases that require several codes for accurate reporting (e.g., spinal fusion with discectomy), hospital-acquired conditions, unspecified codes, and resource-intensive DRGs. Challenges facing effective coding compliance audit programs may include insufficient documentation, insufficient physician queries, difficulties in understanding ICD-10-PCS procedural coding logic, difficulties in understanding how to code multiple complex procedures, misunderstanding of root operation definitions and applications, and failure to code to the highest level of specificity. Despite the challenges, effective coding audit programs are achievable and many opportunities exist going forward to educate and mentor coding professionals to become subject matter experts.

PREBILL AND RETROSPECTIVE CODING AUDITS

A prebill coding audit is an audit that is conducted before the initial claim is ever submitted to the payer. The benefit to conducting a prebill audit is that errors are identified and corrected proactively, which prevents payment denials and/or payment take-backs by the payer. A prebill audit provides an opportunity for the auditor to identify any "red flags," which can alert governmental payers of potential errors through their data analysis software. Prebill audits result in high reimbursement for providers because repetitive paybacks are reduced or eliminated. On the contrary, a retrospective coding audit is performed after the initial claim has been submitted to the payer, and if errors are identified during the audit, a subsequent bill with corrected errors is submitted. This results in extra work effort for the billing department and can raise red flags with payers.

PREBILL CODING AUDITS

Hospitals would be wise to implement prebill inpatient and outpatient coding audits for the purpose of validating diagnosis-related group (DRG) and ambulatory payment classification (APC) assignments before the patient's bill is finalized and submitted to the payer. By doing so, the volume of back-end work decreases and the volume of repeated bill submissions decreases. In other words, if the DRG and/or APC assignments are noted to be correct prior to the bill/claim submission, then there should be fewer resubmissions of claims due to DRG and/or APC errors and fewer claim denials overall. The process of prebill coding audits is simple. High-risk DRGs/APCs can be identified through data analysis, and that information is then passed along to the coders. The coders would then know to submit accounts with the designated high-risk accounts to an auditing queue. The coding auditors would then review all accounts submitted to the queue for accuracy, and upon completion they would return the account to a coding queue for the coder to assess whether the auditor agreed or disagreed. For disagreements, the coder would need to revisit the documentation and consider changing the DRG/APC assignment. If the coder agreed with the auditor's recommendations, then the changes would be made and the claim is finalized. If the coder disagreed with the auditor's recommendations, then the coder would appeal until an agreement between the two parties could be reached. The bill would never be finalized until an agreement was reached.

HEALTH RECORD ELEMENTS SELECTED FOR ABSTRACTION

Coders are responsible for abstracting and verifying certain types of information from a health record. This process is performed as part of creating the final bill. The following elements are typically selected for abstraction and verification:

- Verify that the patient's admit date and discharge dates match the physician's orders.
- Verify that the discharge disposition matches case management notes, discharge summary, physician orders, and/or progress notes.
- Verify that the attending physician matches the physician's name included on the admit order.
- For newborn accounts, enter the birth weight in pounds and ounces or grams, Apgar scores, and number of ventilator days if applicable.
- Enter all consulting physician names, date of consults, and service line.

Diagnostic and procedural code assignments are entered via the encoder process of computing and completing the assignments. After the codes are merged into the abstract from the encoder, the coder should then enter any operative dates, surgeon names, tissue type, anesthesia type, anesthesia doctor, and assistant surgeon names, as applicable. For obstetric accounts, enter the length of labor in hours, number of live births, date of delivery, number of stillborn, and delivery method. For accounts wherein the patient expired, the coder should enter the cause of death as noted on the death summary, final progress note, or emergency room record.

IMPORTANCE OF ABSTRACTING THE APPROPRIATE DISCHARGE DISPOSITION CODE FROM A RECORD

A patient's discharge disposition code assignment can impact reimbursement calculations. It is important for healthcare providers to document in the patient's record the correct disposition code. Examples of disposition codes or discharge destinations that impact reimbursement can be rehabilitation unit, skilled nursing facility, home, or home with home health services. The difference in payment methodologies in correlation to discharge disposition codes is a direct result of Medicare's Post-Acute Care Transformation Act of 2014. Not only does the discharge disposition code affect reimbursement calculations, but it also impacts the severity of illness, risk of mortality, and core measure algorithms. Coders are responsible for selecting the appropriate status from the medical record documentation to include on the final bill. Reliable sources of documentation that coders may reference to determine the appropriate status include case management notes, discharge summary, physician orders, and/or progress notes.

PURPOSE OF AN ENCODER

An encoder is an electronic tool that receives diagnostic or procedural data manually entered by a coder and then converts the data into a numerical code. An encoder is a logic-driven tool that prompts the coder through several choices/options until the appropriate code is achieved. This tool promotes consistency and accuracy because it potentially prevents the coder from missing a

81

key piece of information. In many computer-assisted coding (CAC) programs, the encoder is an integral part. The encoder serves the same purpose in CAC as it does in a stand-alone encoder — logically guide the coder to the appropriate code selection based upon the providers' documentation. Whether a coder uses a stand-alone encoder, a CAC encoder, or codes with an ICD-10 book only, the critical skill for the coder is to accurately and thoroughly search the health information for the diagnoses and procedures that affect the hospital stay.

CAC

CAC is the acronym for computer-assisted coding. CAC software is a helpful aid to coders in that it analyzes electronic health information for specific medical terms and phrases that correlate to numerical codes. CAC software uses natural language processing to identify the terminology. CAC offers many benefits to a coder, such as efficiency in coding, increased production, decrease in average coding turn-around time, consistency in following coding guidelines, and decreased coding error rates. Even though coding errors rates may decrease, it is still imperative for a coder to double-check the CAC-assigned codes because CAC is capable of selecting incorrect terminology. For example, CAC may select cancer as a diagnosis to code, but in reality, the appropriate code should reflect history of cancer.

NLP

Natural language processing (NLP) is an integral and important part of computer-assisted coding (CAC). NLP technology has the capability to process text as well as data fields containing text into suggested ICD-10 codes. NLP technologies differ in how they decipher narrative texts, how they recognize coding-related data, and how they integrate data among systems. An efficient CAC system will be one that correctly suggests accurate codes based upon coding and/or regulatory guidelines, and through the CAC's accuracy, the coder's job is more easily accomplished. In other words, if a CAC-recommended code has supporting documentation and is an accurate recommendation, the coder can review the suggested code and documentation more quickly, thus increasing production. The best CAC system will operate with an NLP with excellent encoder functionality so that the coder does not have to access various systems of an encoder, coding references, electronic health record, etc.

POTENTIAL PROBLEMS WITH CAC-ASSIGNED CODES AND IMPORTANCE OF VALIDATING THOSE CODES

Computer-assisted coding (CAC) software does not diminish the role of a coder. Rather, the value of having the coder's knowledge and skills applied to the CAC process enhances the overall coding accuracy. In other words, coders will not be replaced by a machine because problems do exist with CAC. One potential problem with CAC-assigned codes pertains to the software's inability to logically decipher complicated cases, and therefore it is necessary for a coder to comprehend the coding rules correctly and assign the appropriate code(s). Another known CAC-related problem is with the software's inability to decipher current illnesses versus

82

historical illnesses as well as illnesses related to family diseases versus personal history.

ASPECTS OF THE REVENUE CYCLE FOR WHICH PROVIDERS MUST STAY ABREAST OF CHANGES

The infrastructure of healthcare is a constantly changing landscape, especially when considering the regulatory requirements that govern its functions. The Affordable Care Act, Medicare Access and CHIP Reauthorization Act, and value-based purchasing are all fairly new initiatives that contribute to the changes and the subsequent need for continuing education. ICD-10-CM/-PCS have provided new challenges in the coding realm, and education must be consistently offered for coders, auditors, revenue cycle staff, and clinicians (for documentation purposes) to stay abreast of coding regulations. The National Correct Coding Initiative (NCCI) contains Centers for Medicare & Medicaid Services edits that identify potential improper payments for Healthcare Common Procedure Coding System and Current Procedural Terminology code assignments, so education surrounding NCCI changes is necessary to prevent or reduce improper reimbursement and/or denials. Medicare's national coverage determinations (NCDs) and local coverage determinations (LCDs) change frequently, and education is necessary to stay abreast of medical necessity issues, coding changes, documentation requirements, etc., pertaining to the NCD/LCDs. Of course, Medicare and Medicaid are not the only payers promoting healthcare regulations; commercial/private payers promote their own rules and regulations through contractual agreements; hence, education is necessary for revenue cycle staff to stay informed of these additional requirements.

PRIORITIZATION OF ACCOUNTS RECEIVABLE

Most healthcare entities will manage A/R through automated software modules. The overall purpose of the modules is to collect monies, and most are designed to prioritize those accounts that are within 15 to 30 days post claim submission. A/R aging reports by payer can be generated as frequently as needed and are used to identify possible payment issues. Priority collection criteria can be imbedded in the modules to route the accounts with high dollar values and/or older accounts to staff for the purpose of addressing them more timely. The healthcare entity's policies and procedures should address prioritization of aged accounts for resolution purposes, and this should include the determination of when an account will be converted to self-pay (in the absence of payment from a third-party payer). This should be taken a step further to also determine when an account should be designated as charity care and/or turned over to an external collection agency.

DISTRIBUTION OF ACCOUNTS RECEIVABLE (A/R) AMONG THE REVENUE CYCLE TEAM

Accounts in an A/R status can be distributed among the revenue cycle team members through several methodologies. Accounts could be divided up as follows:

- By the patients' last names assigned to different employees (e.g., last names ending in A–BI may be assigned to employee #1, BJ–CE assigned to employee #2, etc.).
- By account number (e.g., numbers ending in 00–01 assigned to employee #1, 02–03 assigned to employee #2, etc.).
- By payer (e.g., Medicaid accounts assigned to employee #1, Medicare accounts assigned to employee #2, etc.).
- By account age (e.g., accounts aged 15+ days are assigned to employee #1, accounts aged 30+ days are assigned to employee #2, etc.).
- By dollar amount (e.g., total charges $1–$15,000 assigned to employee #1, etc.).
- By an automated queue assignment that assigns accounts to the next ready employee.

It would be expected that management would monitor the assignments regardless of the method of distribution selected because volumes fluctuate and it would be necessary to ensure that some employees are not becoming overwhelmed with too much volume and others with too little volume.

CHARGEMASTER

PURPOSE

A hospital has a database that contains all charges for services rendered. This database is known as the chargemaster or charge description master (CDM). The CDM is the core of a hospital's revenue cycle. Each hospital department is responsible for entering the type of service or supply provided to a patient. Each procedure, supply, or service has its own unique item number. For each charge, a Current Procedural Terminology /Healthcare Common Procedure Coding System code and revenue code as well as other financial elements are assigned. The functions of the CDM are to not only assign charges, but also to produce itemized statements, produce a valid claim, monitor costs, and generate financial reporting.

ELEMENTS

A hospital's chargemaster is composed of certain key elements. The typical data elements could be the following:

- Charge description: Each charge has a title that describes the charge whether it is a supply, a medication, a procedure, etc.
- Current Procedural Terminology (CPT)/Healthcare Common Procedure Coding System (HCPCS) code and modifiers: A CPT or HCPCS code may be assigned to a specific procedure or supply, and applicable modifiers may be built in to the charge as well. Of note, not all charges will have a corresponding CPT/HCPCS code or modifier.

84

- Revenue code: This is a three-digit number that represents the location of the patient when the service was rendered or the type of service that the patient received.
- Charge dollar amount: This is the cost associated with the service or supply provided.
- Charge code: This is the unique number assigned to each item listed in the chargemaster. It is also known as the charge description master number.
- Charge status: This represents whether or not the charge has been allocated to the patient's account and its payment or denial status.

MEDICARE ENROLLMENT PROCESS FOR PHYSICIANS

Physicians have a choice of whether or not to enroll in the Medicare program and thus be eligible to receive Medicare payment for services rendered to Medicare beneficiaries. There is a required enrollment application process that physicians must complete in order to be eligible. The application, and later any changes to enrollment, may be completed through an Internet-based system known as the Provider Enrollment, Chain, and Ownership System. Providers must also submit a participation agreement along with the Medicare enrollment form. The participation agreement states that the provider will accept assignment of claims for all services provided to Medicare beneficiaries, which means the provider accepts the Medicare-allowed amount as full payment. It also means that the provider cannot collect more monies from the beneficiary through deductibles or coinsurance. The National Provider Identifier (NPI) number must be included in the enrollment application and participation agreement. As part of the credentialing process, healthcare entities should ask providers for their NPI number as well as proof of Medicare participation.

CMI

The case mix index (CMI) is a metric watched closely by healthcare administrators. It is an indicator of the healthcare patient population's severity of illness. It serves as the basis for payment methodologies. It can also serve as a barometer of adequate or inadequate diagnosis-related group (DRG) assignments, meaning that if the CMI value is low, then the DRGs may not adequately reflect the severity of illness and the associated resource expenditures. CMI values can be calculated for individual providers, service lines, entire hospitals, and/or payers. The CMI value is calculated by adding the relative weights (RWs) (for a defined time period) and then dividing the sum by the number of patients (e.g., RW 0.65, RW 0.70, RW 1.25 = 2.6/3 patients = 0.87 CMI). The RWs of a DRG impact the CMI value; the higher the RW, the higher the CMI.

Compliance

AGENCY FOR HEALTHCARE RESEARCH AND QUALITY'S PATIENT SAFETY INDICATORS

The Agency for Healthcare Research and Quality's mission is to measure outcomes and produce evidence to make healthcare safer and of higher quality. Patient safety indicators (PSIs) are indicators that provide information regarding complications and/or adverse effects. PSIs help hospitals identify complications and/or adverse effects that are in need of further research and that may affect patient safety. Some examples of PSIs are PSI 03, pressure ulcer rate; PSI 06, iatrogenic pneumothorax rate; PSI 08, postoperative hip fracture rate; and PSI 09, postoperative hemorrhage or hematoma rate. Clinical documentation improvement specialists are instrumental in the capture of PSIs. The PSI information that is captured is then used in national performance measures pertaining to patient safety. The purpose of identifying and sharing PSI information is to keep patients safe from medical errors. PSI data are collected and used to rate hospitals according to performance measures regarding safety.

JOINT COMMISSION'S NPSGs

The Joint Commission's National Patient Safety Goals (NPSGs) address certain areas of concern regarding patient safety in healthcare. The Joint Commission is responsible for developing and updating the NPSG annually. Examples of NPSG goals are as follows:

- Improve the accuracy of patient identification, accomplished through the use of at least two patient identifiers when providing treatment.
- Improve communication among healthcare providers through the reporting of critical results in a timely manner.
- Improve the safety of medication use by labeling all medications, containers, and solutions that are used in procedural settings.
- Reduce the risk of healthcare-acquired infections through compliance with the Centers for Disease Control and Prevention's guidance pertaining to handwashing techniques and through the use of evidence-based practices to prevent catheter-associated bloodstream infections or urinary tract infections.
- Reduce the risk of falls, and prevent the development of pressure ulcers in the healthcare setting.

PROCESS IMPROVEMENT PLAN COMPONENTS

Process improvement plans should include the following components:

- An abstract or summary of the overall plan.
- Approvals by responsible parties.
- Revision history of the plan to include the revision number, release date, author's name, and reason for the change(s).
- Purpose of the document.

- Definitions of key terms, acronyms, and abbreviations.
- Cited references or resources.
- Plan overview to include the scope, goals, and objectives.
- Key stakeholders and their roles and responsibilities in the project.
- Critical success factors.
- Assumptions about the plan.
- Constraints of the plan.
- Risks that may have a negative impact upon the plan.
- Tracking of risks and issues and logs pertaining to the risks and issues.
- Status reporting throughout the various phases of the plan.
- Implementation phase to introduce the project to the organization.
- Training requirements.
- Project deliverables and repository.
- Project schedule and key milestones.

TREND ANALYSIS FOR IMPROVEMENT PLANNING

Trend analysis is a key function in identifying variations of current performance in comparison to past performances, and it may predict future performance. Trend analysis is an excellent tool to assist in performance improvement plans and initiatives. For example, a hospital may monitor its mortality rates, morbidity rates, complication rates, and efficiency rates over several years' time. The hospital may compare or benchmark their own rates against the rates of other hospitals' Medicare data within the state, MedPAR data, and/or CareScience data. MedPAR consolidates claims data from the Centers for Medicare & Medicaid Services' National Claims History files. Hospitals, on a quarterly basis, can review their MedPAR trend data in comparison to state and national results, seeing exactly where their billing/coding data fall above or below averages. This information can then be used in developing performance improvement plans.

RISK ANALYSIS AND RISK MANAGEMENT IN HEALTHCARE

Healthcare risk analysis and risk management are based upon the Centers for Medicare & Medicaid Services (CMS)'s Security Rule for the protection of electronic protected health information (e-PHI). CMS's Security Rule requires that all e-PHI be kept secure from vulnerabilities in each healthcare entity's environment, and that policies and procedures address risks, threats, and vulnerabilities. Risk management staff should include IT and health information management (HIM) representatives to address the security of e-PHI. These individuals would need to be involved in risk analysis procedures, and the risk analysis procedures would include identification of the analysis scope, data collection, identification of threats and vulnerabilities, assessment of current security measures, assessment of threat occurrence and impact, identification of security measures, and documentation procedures. The Security Rule requires risk analyses to be documented, and the documentation to then be used in the risk management process. The risk management process includes development of a plan, implementation of security measures, and evaluation and maintenance of security measures. Documentation of

87

security plans and measures may also be requested by external auditors for review; HIM, IT, and risk management personnel should collaborate regarding documentation submission for these external requests.

ANNUAL RISK ASSESSMENT

It is wise for healthcare compliance and audit departments to incorporate an annual risk assessment into their management plans. The risk assessment would be the first step in the development of the annual audit plan. An audit plan cannot be designed without the knowledge of where the healthcare system's risks lie. The risk assessment process has multiple layers that include interviews of administrative and departmental management; surveys; review of new federal regulations (e.g., Office of Inspector General's fiscal year audit plan); and review of previous audit plans, specifically any unaddressed audits. Once information is gathered from these sources, it should be analyzed and categorized into the appropriate section of the audit universe. Scoring of each risk would be the next step. Scoring involves assessing the likelihood of material impact and the loss of confidence associated with the risk. Once scoring is complete, those risks with the highest scores would most likely be included in the upcoming fiscal year's audit plan.

ENTITIES THAT REGULATE HEALTHCARE DIRECTLY AND INDIRECTLY

Enterprise risk management (ERM) is a process in which a healthcare entity's administrative personnel and board of directors identify potential events that may adversely affect the entity and then manage the risk to provide assurance that the entity's objectives will be achieved. Part of ERM is to identify which external entities regulate their healthcare entity directly and/or indirectly. These external entities will include (at a minimum): Congress, the federal circuit courts, Supreme Court, Centers for Medicare & Medicaid Services, Office of Inspector General, Department of Justice, quality improvement organizations, recovery audit contractors, Medicaid independent contractors, Medicare administrative contractors, durable medical equipment contractors, Internal Revenue Service, Office for Civil Rights, Occupational Safety and Health Administration, Federal Drug Administration, U.S. Department of Health and Human Services, Federal Bureau of Investigations, Environmental Protection Agency, Health Resources and Services Administration, the Joint Commission, state Medicaid, state surveys, state departments of public health, state medical boards, state nursing boards, and state licensure.

MEDICAL IDENTITY THEFT

Medical identity theft is on the rise. The impact upon patients can be devastating because the breach may result in criminals maximizing health benefits of the victim's insurance plan, or the criminal may be successful in obtaining prescription drugs. In some cases, thieves hold health information ransom, demanding large sums of money to return the health information to the patient or healthcare entity. Health information management (HIM) professionals should be involved in mitigating the risks associated with medical identity theft. HIM professionals can build awareness that medical identity is a patient safety issue. They can provide staff education regarding how to identify fraudulent activity. They can work with

88

information technology personnel in mitigating phishing scams and initiating valid passcode applications. HIM professionals can assist in identifying fraudulent activity through data analysis and the performance of proactive audits.

The Centers for Medicare & Medicaid Services (CMS) is well aware of medical identity theft and the various techniques that thieves are using to steal information. CMS is especially concerned with one particular piece of information that thieves target, which is Social Security numbers. An effective deterrent that is being actively pursued is the removal of the Social Security number from the Medicare/Medicaid card. The new Medicare Access and CHIP Reauthorization Act requires the U.S. Department of Health and Human Services to collaborate with the commissioner of Social Security to ensure that Social Security numbers are not included on the card. This is also known as the Social Security Number Removal Initiative. By 2018, the card will include a randomly assigned Medicare beneficiary identifier (MBI) instead of a Social Security number. The new MBI must be used in all healthcare interactions. This initiative will minimize the risk of identity theft for Medicare/Medicaid beneficiaries. In consideration of this initiative, health information management professionals should be involved in healthcare policy revisions regarding whether or not Social Security numbers should even be collected going forward. If it is determined the Social Security number is still needed, then HIM professionals should assist with determining how it will be stored and who will have access to it.

MEDICAL IDENTITY THEFT RESPONSE PROGRAM

When a medical identity theft incident occurs, the healthcare entity must promptly respond. As part of the program requirements, patients affected by identity theft must be notified of the incident. The privacy officer, health information management department, financial accounting, and involved physicians should be notified. A faux medical record should be created that includes the thief's information. The affected patient and possibly involved physicians would need to be involved in this process to identify what information is accurate and what information is false (fabricated by the thief). Both patient records would need to be flagged indefinitely in order to alert all healthcare providers of the medical identity theft incident. A final step in the program should be that the healthcare entity offers the victim free credit and/or medical identity monitoring services. This service should be provided for a minimum of three years.

INVESTIGATIVE METHODS

When notification from a consumer reporting agency of a medical identity theft incident has occurred, a medical theft response team should act promptly. The master patient index should be referenced for accuracy of Social Security number, driver's license number, U.S. passport, legal permanent resident card, telephone number, address, etc., aiming to identify discrepancies between the new information and information already on file. Patient signatures on file can be compared to signatures on new documents, looking specifically for signs of forgery. Discrepancies in the spelling of the patient's name, birth date, and/or clinical information (such as height or weight), can be clues of a possible identity theft, as well as invalid addresses and phone numbers. Naturally, if a new patient submits information during registration that is confirmed as belonging to a deceased individual, there should be immediate concerns of attempted identity theft.

CODING COMPLIANCE

Coding compliance is an important function of healthcare operations secondary to federal regulations. Code assignments must be supported by clinical documentation in order to avoid denials by payers and/or appeal their decisions. Discrepancies between coded data and supporting documentation can be identified through data analytics and/or through internal auditing processes. Through the auditing of records identified as high-risk accounts (based on diagnosis-related groups), internal auditors identify documentation insufficiencies/discrepancies. For example, a coder assigns the principal diagnosis as lung mass. However, upon closer inspection of the medical record documentation, the internal auditor finds documentation of lung carcinoma with metastases to the mediastinal lymph nodes. Both diagnoses have corresponding codes that the coder missed entirely, and both diagnoses and their corresponding codes correlate to a positive financial impact.

TRENDING CODING COMPLIANCE DATA

Healthcare administration will expect to receive information (daily, monthly, or quarterly) pertaining to coding compliance. Each healthcare entity will need to decide upon what coding compliance data should be collected, the frequency of its collection, and the reasoning behind its collection. This should be acknowledged through policies and procedures. The importance of collecting and trending coding compliance data is understood to impact (either directly or indirectly) clinical and financial decision making. Examples of coding compliance data that should be collected are as follows (this list is not exhaustive):

- Diagnosis-related group (DRG) assignment accuracy.
- Present-on-admission indicator assignment accuracy.
- Discharge disposition assignment accuracy.
- Principal diagnosis code assignment accuracy.
- Principal procedure code assignment accuracy.
- Validation of attending physician and surgeon names assigned in the abstract.
- Coding and/or auditing productivity.

Measuring the productivity of coding audits, the coding compliance accuracy rates, and the associated overall net financial impact can be used in a cost-benefit analysis to support additional staff acquisitions. For example, if two coding auditors yield a net financial impact (based on DRG changes resulting from the audits) of $1 million annually, then further calculations can be conducted to illustrate the projected monetary gain if more coding auditors were to be hired.

Effective Coding Educational Program

Healthcare entities should implement a coding compliance educational program. The components of such a program should include the following:

- Promotion of coding guidelines.
- Promotion of federal regulations.
- Development of policies and procedures pertaining to coding education.
- Demonstration of the healthcare entity's commitment to coding compliance to all stakeholders.

Coding educational efforts should apply to both new and established coding personnel. New coding personnel should go through a "ramp-up" process, meaning they are progressed through stages of advancement over time (e.g., production at 3 months = 50%, 4 months = 75%, etc. and quality measures at 3 months = 85%, 4 months = 90%, etc.). Educational needs should be reassessed annually. Various means of educational delivery should be offered to coding personnel, such as face-to-face meetings, webinars, module learning, etc. Examples of types of education that should be offered to new employees and readdressed with established employees may include evaluation and management (E/M) coding, modifier usage, Current Procedural Terminology (CPT) coding, ICD-10 coding, excisional debridements, interventional radiology, sepsis, etc.

NCCI

The National Correct Coding Initiative (NCCI) was developed by the Centers for Medicare & Medicaid Services for the purpose of encouraging correct coding methodologies nationwide. NCCI is applicable to Part B claims only. Healthcare entities can assess their coding accuracy prior to submitting a Part B claim and thus potentially prevent an inappropriate payment and/or a denial. NCCI edits (also known as Procedure-to-Procedure code pair edits) can provide the guidance needed to assess coding accuracy. Additionally, there are medically unlikely edits, which identify the maximum number of units that can be billed for a single code. All of these measures aid the coder/biller in preventing inappropriate code combinations.

Involvement in Resolving NCCI Edits

Certified coders, who are knowledgeable in proper coding methodologies, should be involved in the workflow process of reconciling any National Correct Coding Initiative (NCCI) edits. An NCCI edit is an indication that at least one code in the code pair is incorrect. Therefore, in such a scenario, the coder can reference the medical record documentation and determine what coding corrections are needed. Coders may be able to identify any inaccurate charges assigned by the various hospital departments, or they may be able to make recommendations for chargemaster changes in order to remain in compliance with coding regulations.

Modifiers Allowed with the NCCI Edits

Modifiers may be appended to a Current Procedural Terminology code so that a CCI edit can be bypassed. Bypassing an edit, however, should only be done if the clinical documentation supports the addition of the modifier. The NCCI edit table will indicate whether the application of a modifier is allowed or not (0 = no modifiers allowed, 1 = modifiers allowed). Anatomical modifiers (e.g., F1, F2, etc.), surgical modifiers (e.g., 25, 58, etc.), and other modifiers (e.g., XE, XP, etc.) are allowed, again depending upon guidance per code in the edit table.

MEDICARE CODE EDITS FOR ICD-10-PCS CODES

For ICD-10-CM/-PCS codes, Medicare has code edits in place to assist with coding accuracy. Some Medicare code edits are listed as follows:

- Invalid diagnosis or procedure code — each code is compared against a table of valid codes, and if a submitted code does not match a code in the table, it is considered invalid.
- Age conflict — If a diagnosis or procedure code is clinically impossible, an edit identifies the conflict. There are four recognized age groups in ICD-10 — newborn, pediatric, adult, and maternity.
- Gender/Sex conflict with the code.
- Noncovered procedure — Medicare does not provide coverage for all procedures.
- Procedure with limited coverage — Medicare limits reimbursement for some procedures that have associated extraordinary costs.

EVALUATING HEALTH INFORMATION MANAGEMENT APPLICATIONS OR TOOLS

When evaluating the efficacy of a health information management application or tool, there are several elements to consider or questions to ask about the application/tool. The following are some examples for consideration:

- Is the application/tool streamlined and without distractions?
- Does it help to accomplish goals and objectives?
- Does it promote a logical sequence of events/workflow?
- Does it allow for multiple ways to express and engage the user, or does it promote limited end results?
- Is it user friendly?
- Will training and/or continuing education be necessary for the users short term or long term?
- What is the average length of time for a user to use the application/tool with ease?
- What is its associated cost?
- Are there any hidden costs?
- Is there free support offered with its use?
- Is there a means to enhance the application/tool as needs change or new demands arise?
- Does it interface with other applications without error?

EHR Vendor Assessment

When considering the selection of an electronic health record (EHR) system, the following steps should be considered. To begin the process, an assessment of the healthcare entity's needs should be performed. This would include identifying EHR features that meet its needs as well as achieve meaningful use. Next, EHR goals should be established. The goals should be specific, measurable, attainable, and on a time schedule. To narrow the vendor choices, a list of "must haves" in an EHR system and "deal breakers" should be determined. To further narrow the field, review certified EHR lists to assist in the decision-making process. These certified lists will note EHR systems that have been tested and approved by the Office of the National Coordinator for Health Information Technology. It is also a good idea to interview colleagues regarding their EHR experiences and research potential vendors' products online prior to the initiation of sales discussions. Demonstrations of EHR products is an essential step in the process, and it is vitally important to ask questions during (and after) the demonstration. Ask vendors for contact names at facilities where a successful EHR implementation has occurred, so that references can be checked and on-site viewings can be scheduled. Finally, compare several vendors' offers to determine the best fit for your healthcare entity.

Computer System or Network System Maintenance

To keep a computer system running properly, system maintenance is necessary. System maintenance may imply network maintenance, physical repair of servers, replacement of servers, or software updates. The primary purpose of conducting computer or system maintenance is to correct defects and enhance performance. Maintenance should also include ensuring that all security updates have been installed. This would include updating all virus protection files, running virus scans, and scanning for malware. Verification that firewalls are working properly is important as well. For maintenance on individual computers, it is important to assess memory capacity and defrag and optimize the hard drive. Maintenance should be performed on a regular basis, and usually it is completed during off-peak hours in order to prevent workflow interruptions. Backup of data is an essential component of maintenance schedules, and most backups are done on a daily basis.

Troubleshooting HIM Software Issues

A well-known, inevitable fact in the health information management (HIM) world is that software will malfunction. Before contacting the information technology (IT) department for assistance, HIM professionals may choose to try the following troubleshooting tips: Close other software programs: This action frees up random access memory, which in turn, can allow the open software to run faster and without glitches. Software can also be shut down and restarted, which may result in resolution of the problem. If a restart of the software does not resolve the problem, then, many times, a reboot of the computer will. Once the computer has rebooted, open the software program again to determine if the glitch is resolved. Use the Internet to search for common errors and their associated remedies. Various forums exist online that contain a data repository of questions, issues, problems, and resolutions that are free for public viewing. If updates to software have recently occurred, there may be a conflict with other software or hardware on the computer. Undoing recent updates or changes may fix the problem or at least provide insight into the root cause of the problem. Viruses, malware, and/or firewall conflicts may prevent proper functioning of software. Removal of viruses/malware and/or changes in firewall settings could resolve software issues. If all else fails, IT is just a phone call away.

HEALTHCARE COMPLIANCE AUDIT

There are multiple types of healthcare compliance audits being conducted in the present day. To understand the purpose of a compliance audit, one must understand the different types of audits. Hospitals should be prepared in the following areas (at a minimum) where audits are likely to occur: Health Insurance Portability and Accountability Act, meaningful use, provider-based status, outlier payments, Medicare's "two-midnight" rule, inpatient claims for mechanical ventilation, ambulatory surgery centers payment system, anesthesia services, outpatient rehabilitation services, immunosuppressive drug claims, hospice, and home health services. The list of potential audits by external agencies is extensive. The Office of Inspector General publishes a work plan for each fiscal year, and this plan is an excellent indicator of where hospitals, skilled nursing facilities, pharmacies, clinics, etc., should focus their attention for internal auditing. The purpose behind each of these external auditors is essentially to identify fraud, waste, and abuse. External auditors will look for opportunities to improve healthcare efficiency, and in many cases, this includes holding accountable those who violate federal healthcare laws.

PREPARING FOR EXTERNAL AUDITS

Hospitals experience audits from external agencies on a regular basis. The external auditors may be representatives of various federal agencies (e.g., Office of Inspector General, the Department of Justice, Medicare administrative contractors). They may represent commercial insurers (e.g., Blue Cross/Blue Shield). The types of audits requested may pertain to charges (e.g., pharmaceutical, supplies, etc.), coding, medical necessity, fraud, contracts, and policies. Preparation should include the development and implementation of policies and procedures, organizational education regarding each department's responsibility during an audit, identification of individuals internally who should be involved in the audits, and determination of appeals processes.

GOVERNMENTAL AUDITS

Federal auditors have the authority to review Medicare and Medicaid claims submitted by providers. Some of federal government audit entities are Medicare recovery audit contractors (RACs), Office of Inspector General (OIG), zone program integrity contractors (ZPICs), and the Department of Justice (DOJ). Depending upon the entity involved, the auditor will have different scopes of work. Also, the number of accounts reviewed, timeline of the audit, and appeals process will vary among the auditors. A RAC's goal is to reduce Medicare improper payments. The focus of the OIG, DOJ, and ZPICs is upon fraud and abuse. Therefore, it is imperative that healthcare organizations be prepared for governmental audits.

EMTALA Audit

EMTALA is the acronym for the Emergency Medical Treatment and Labor Act. Congress enacted EMTALA in 1986 to ensure that all people would have access to emergency services regardless of the individual's ability to pay. This act mandates hospitals to provide stabilizing treatment for a patient with an emergency medical condition, and if it is unable to stabilize the patient, the hospital is required to transfer the patient to a facility where stabilization can occur. EMTALA is enforced by the Centers for Medicare & Medicaid Services as well as the Office of Inspector General (OIG), and either entity may conduct an audit. To prepare for an EMTALA audit, hospitals should review their EMTALA and transfer policies and procedures (P&Ps), medical staff bylaws, physician on-call lists, emergency workflows, emergency department transfer form, and emergency department signage. P&Ps should be up to date with EMTALA guidelines. Medical staff bylaws should indicate who is allowed to perform the medical screening exam. The emergency workflow should be EMTALA compliant, and signage should be easy to understand and follow from the patient's perspective. The transfer forms must be completed in their entirety, and on-call lists must correspond with documentation in the medical record.

Leadership

POLICIES AND PROCEDURES

KEY ELEMENTS

Healthcare organizations should follow policy and procedure guidelines and templates and/or specified formats. The following are the key elements to include in policy and procedures:

- Title (representing the subject or topic).
- Reference number for tracking purposes.
- Statement of purpose.
- Regulatory citations and/or external references.
- Scope that defines resources.
- Effective date as well as revision dates.
- Administrative approval signatures.
- Policy statement that identifies measurable objectives, responsible parties, and monitoring of compliance.
- Detailed procedural steps.

WRITING EFFECTIVE POLICIES AND PROCEDURES

Effective policies and procedures should be written with key essential elements. The policy statement should include measurable objectives, designation of responsibilities, and monitoring methods to ensure compliance. Policy statements are written at a broad, high level. They should be written in compliance with associated regulatory guidance to the topic at hand. Procedures outline the detailed steps for the designated responsible party to follow in order to carry out tasks. Procedural steps should list any resources and/or tools needed to follow the step. The steps should outline where the work will occur, what equates to a completed step, how communication will occur between involved parties, what supportive documentation will be required, and how results will be maintained and/or stored.

MANAGEMENT

A robust policy and procedure (P&P) program is an absolute necessity in the ever-changing healthcare landscape of federal and statutory regulations, Centers for Medicare & Medicaid Services regulations, Joint Commission standards, and multiple other accreditation bodies and compliance enforcers. No longer is it feasible for P&Ps to exist in a decentralized manner of three-ring notebook binders. The sheer volume of electronic information alone mandates up-to-date, available, and effective P&Ps. This requires management to pay close attention to ensuring that P&Ps are current. Technology is an excellent tool to streamline the management of P&Ps. A web-based system of P&P management is an excellent method to control and update the process and disseminate effective P&Ps. In other words, automation allows for version control and promotes ease and efficiency in locating up-to-date documents.

Implementation of an automated centralized policy and procedure (P&P) program may provide ease of access for employees to attain the most current version of a P&P, but ensuring that the employee(s) understands the content is another area of concern. First, it is important to determine which employees have read the P&Ps. Through an automated database, access to P&Ps can be assessed by analyzing audit trails. An audit trail reveals who opened a document and if the individual accepted the policy and when. Tests can subsequently be distributed to employees to assess their comprehension of the content. If testing reveals a lack of comprehension, then further training can be provided until a level of acceptable comprehension results is achieved. Audit trails and testing results provide concrete evidence of compliance; therefore, it is important for management to maintain such documents.

SELECTING AN EHR SYSTEM

When selecting an electronic health record (EHR) system, significant planning will be a reality. One of the best ways to begin the process is to identify the healthcare entity's key goals and then select an EHR system that meets the key goals. Most healthcare entities will choose to go with a vendor's EHR system instead of building their own. Therefore, it will be necessary to ensure that the vendor's system will meet the established key goals for the healthcare entity. Pricing of the EHR system should be clarified in the beginning stages and should include costs associated with hardware, software, maintenance, interfacing/networking charges, connection costs to health information exchange platforms, etc. Data migration will be a significant component of EHR implementation; therefore, significant planning must be conducted to determine which data will migrate and how much data will migrate, and the location of the data or data templates should be determined. Integration with other products must be considered upfront to ensure a successful implementation and reduce risks of adverse events (e.g., inability to bill, inability to access essential data, etc.). It is to be expected that health information management personnel will participate in this entire process.

SDLC

The systems development life cycle (SDLC) refers to the development or modification of an information system or information database. The planning phase of the SDLC begins with a project request submitted to a steering committee. The steering committee reviews all requests, allocates resources for the approved requests, and develops a project development team for the approved project. During the analysis phase of the SDLC, a feasibility study is conducted along with a detailed analysis, both aimed at determining the exact problem or improvement opportunity. A system proposal will occur next in the life cycle, and this proposal will recommend feasible solutions for the project to the steering committee who will then decide how the system will be developed. Possible solutions may be to purchase software or create customized software or outsource services. This leads into the design phase with the acquisition of hardware and/or software followed by the testing of products for performance reliability. A mockup form may be created to input or output actual data to determine its accuracy and reliability, and this may be

97

followed by the development of a prototype. The implementation phase of the SDLC occurs next with conversion to the new system and training opportunities for users, followed by the support phase, which provides ongoing assistance after implementation.

END-USER NEEDS ANALYSIS PROCESS

An end-user needs analysis process can be divided into three phases: (1) preparation, (2) investigation, and (3) decision.

1. In the preparation phase, one would identify the problem, evaluation criteria, stakeholders, and goals. Problems may lie in workflow structures, organizational structure, limited resources, or technical issues.
2. In the investigative phase, one would determine the present situation and the desired future situation. This would involve reviewing workflow diagrams, network patterns, mapping of information pathways, and/or narrative descriptions of the existing system. It is also important in this step to understand what end users think that the problem(s) may be. To progress to a future desired state, the investigative process would need to consider adding or changing resources or upgrading to systems with new features.
3. In the decision phase, one would propose a model for implementation, and then the decision would need to be made as to whether to build it in house or purchase it from a vendor. A model should include the pros and cons of recommended changes, outlining optimal solutions that are the most feasible with the lowest associated costs. A cost-benefit analysis would be beneficial for consideration in this phase.

DETERMINING AUDIT CRITERIA

Before an audit can begin, the auditor must determine specific criteria to follow. The criteria help to develop the framework of the audit and keep the auditor organized and away from scope creep. An organizational risk assessment begins the audit process through the identification of risks (i.e., regulatory, financial, etc.) and their potential impact for the entity. Once risks are identified and scored according to a range from highest to lowest risks, then an annual audit plan is developed. The audit plan determines which specific hospital departments need to be audited and why those departments need to be audited. Determination of what needs to be audited may be based upon regulatory guidance and/or administrative guidance. The timing of audits may depend upon regulatory deadlines, merger acquisitions and the transfer of data, and/or administrative requests. The mechanics of how the audit should be conducted must rely upon international audit standards and auditors' ethical standards.

WORKFLOW

A workflow is the logical progression of steps for the purpose of accomplishing tasks, through the process of passing along data or information to a participant for further action, in compliance with pre-established procedural rules. Healthcare organization use workflows to coordinate tasks between individuals or departments

98

and ultimately accomplish procedural efficiency, procedural compliance, cost savings, and transparency (through visible audit trails). There are three different types of workflows: sequential (similar to flowcharts), state machine (more complex, returning to a previous step if needed), and rules-driven (the rules determine the progress of the workflow). Workflow software (e.g., SharePoint) offers many benefits, such as improved productivity, transparency, faster turnaround times, improved accountability, cost savings, and reductions in error rates.

WORKFLOW ANALYSIS

Workflow analysis is the process of reviewing all steps in a workflow to identify inefficiencies and then recommend improvement opportunities. The analysis process involves meeting with the "owners" of the workflow to gain an understanding of their current process, any known problems/issues, and their desired outcome. Continuous process improvement should be sought after by healthcare entities especially in light of technological advancements and constant change. Workflow analysis can take into account these changes and make recommendations on how to improve workflows to be more efficient and less costly. A large portion of workflow analysis includes interviewing key individuals involved in the workflow. This would include those who are involved at the beginning of the workflow process and extend to those at the end of the workflow. Documentation of each workflow step is key to identifying inefficiencies and identifying opportunities for improvement. Once the analysis is completed, the results are typically presented to lower level management to ensure that they are accurate and realistic. After adjustments are made, the final recommendations are made to the administration for consideration.

DEVELOPING A WORKFLOW PROCESS

A workflow process specifies the order of execution of the flow of work. Conditions that must be accomplished should be incorporated into the design to route the tasks either through a sequential, alternative, parallel, or iterative process. Another way of describing this process is to refer to it as a flow diagram. Sequential routing is the simplest process in that it proceeds from point A to point B and so on, without alternate pathways. Conditional routing considers a task and then follows the task with at least two options before reaching the next step (e.g., task A followed by either option B or C with either choice resulting in step D). Parallel routing considers a task and then follows the task with two required choices before reaching the next step (e.g., task A followed by both option B and C and both options resulting in step D). Iterative routing considers a task and then flows to the next two steps with the latter step possibly repeating back to the previous step and eventually reaching the final step (e.g., task A followed by task B followed by task C, which may repeat back to task B and task C before resulting in task D).

99

DESIGNING ELECTRONIC HEALTH INFORMATION MANAGEMENT WORKFLOW PROCESSES

When designing an electronic health information management workflow, it is important to first understand basic workflow logic. One step in a workflow process can perform multiple actions if designed to do so. Workflow processes should be designed so that they flow logically from the previous step. If a step in the flow contains only actions and no conditions, then the workflow will perform the designated actions. If a step includes conditions, then the step can only be satisfied when the conditions are met. A workflow must be hyperlinked or attached to a preexisting database, list, or library; if there are no preexisting resources, then a new resource must be created. To complete a newly designed workflow, the final step is to test the process before publishing, and if an error exists (such as a break in a hyperlink), then error symbols will appear next to each step for the parameter that is invalid. Measures will then need to be taken to correct the errors.

ORGANIZING DATA IN INTRADEPARTMENTAL WORKFLOW DESIGN

When designing intradepartmental workflows, it is necessary to organize data in a logical manner. An example of creating a workflow between departments could be organized around coding audit functions. Once the coded accounts are added to an audit queue, the auditor would be responsible for adding accounts to an audit database for review. The audit database should be organized according to account number, date of service, coder name, auditor name, pertinent diagnostic and procedural codes, diagnosis-related group (DRG) and/or ambulatory payment classification (APC) assignment, and accuracy rates. If, after review, the accuracy rates of code assignments and/or DRG/APC assignments are 100%, then the account would cease to move in the workflow design. If the accuracy rate(s) were less than 100%, the accounts should move to the coder's queue for their assessment of the auditor's recommendations. If in agreement, codes and/or DRG/APC assignments would be corrected, and then the account would move to the billing department for a rebill. If not in agreement, an appeal would be issued by the coder with movement of the account back to the auditor for a second review. If the appeal was rejected, then managerial staff should be involved for final determination. All of the back-and-forth flow of accounts cannot function appropriately without efficient data organization in the database.

LIFELONG LEARNING FOR CODERS

Lifelong learning is an absolute must for coders for many reasons. Annually, changes are made to ICD-10-CM/PCS codes as well as Current Procedural Terminology codes, which dictate coder education. Frequent changes are made to coding guidelines and federal regulations, which also dictate coder education. Keeping up to speed on regulatory changes may require review of new and/or revised national and/or local coverage determinations and payer policies. Technological advances in healthcare happen often, which forces coders to learn the new procedures in order to understand correct code assignment. Coder professional development can also be in the form composing and presenting coding topics to their local component state association and/or other coding publications.

BALANCED WORKLOADS AMONG TEAM MEMBERS

Whether the task at hand is coding, auditing, release of information, or deficiency analysis, the volume of tasks can be overwhelming to health information management teams. It is therefore essential for management to implement an annual workload distribution plan that is reassessed periodically (e.g., monthly, quarterly, etc.). It is also essential for management to assess and rebalance daily workload volumes to ensure that tasks are completed on schedule and that team members are not overloaded. Management should be familiar with each team member's skill set to ensure that employees are functioning at their highest level of knowledge, experience, abilities, and skills. If the assessment reveals weaknesses in certain areas, then responsibilities should be shifted to other team members who can better excel in that area of responsibility. Management should request feedback from each team member as to their opinion of where the workload may be imbalanced. Communication between management and team members is key to an effective workload distribution plan, and discussions should be held on at least a weekly basis.

DELEGATING WORKLOAD ASSIGNMENTS

The process of delegating workload assignments should include the following considerations:

- Determination of the task(s) to be delegated and to what resource or role the task(s) should be assigned.
- Determination of which employee triggers the delegation (e.g., an employee whose role is associated with the task(s) or a supervisor responsible for the task(s).
- Determination of why the delegation is triggered (e.g., an employee who is on vacation, out sick, or overloaded in their daily assignments; an approaching deadline; or lack of performance).
- Determination of the turnaround time frame (e.g., a specific calendar date, by week's end, or prior to a vacation).

Each of these delegation dimensions must be considered in order for implementation of workloads to be efficient and effective.

RHIT Practice Test

1. A laboratory test is intended to measure the incidence of cancer cells in a particular sample, but instead, it determines the number of healthy cells. Which characteristic of this laboratory test is deficient?

    a. Validity
    b. Reliability
    c. Specificity
    d. Sensitivity

2. What is typically the first step in a progressive disciplinary process?

    a. Written reprimand
    b. Termination
    c. Suspension
    d. Oral warning

3. Which of the following pieces of data must be collected during each visit to a health practitioner?

    a. Ethnicity
    b. Date of birth
    c. Name
    d. Self-reported health status

4. During the month of January, a 400-bed health care facility had 450 deaths, 2,500 other discharges, and 11,000 inpatient service days. What was the inpatient bed occupancy rate for January? Round to the nearest percentage point.

    a. 44%
    b. 28%
    c. 89%
    d. 94%

5. An organization surveys the members of a community about their alcohol consumption. Questionnaires are mailed to the local residents along with self-addressed stamped envelopes. The results of the survey indicate that the area has a below-average rate of alcoholism. What is the most likely reason for these results?

    a. Diagnosis bias
    b. Nonresponse bias
    c. Prevarication bias
    d. Survival bias

6. A health care administrator, looking for ways to decrease patient wait time in the emergency room, studies the methods successful restaurants have used to increase table turnover. What quality improvement strategy is the administrator using?

a. Internal benchmarking
b. Performance benchmarking
c. Comparative benchmarking
d. Competitive benchmarking

7. Which form of management makes the most use of statistical analysis?

a. Risk management
b. Utilization management
c. Participatory management
d. Quality assessment

8. Which coding instrument is generally recommended for the principal diagnosis upon admittance to inpatient treatment?

a. SNOMED
b. ICD-10-CM
c. DSM-5
d. HCPCS

9. Which piece of legislation created a program for detecting fraudulent health plans?

a. Health Insurance Portability and Accountability Act of 1996
b. Nursing Home Reform Act of 1987
c. Patient Self-Determination Act of 1990
d. Consolidated Omnibus Budget Reconciliation Act of 1995

10. Which of the following is a basic assumption of normative decision theory?

a. Decision makers can never fully understand their situations.
b. Decision makers cannot maximize revenue.
c. Decision makers tend toward satisfying choices.
d. Decision makers have total knowledge of the available options.

11. A health care administrator is establishing budgets for staff. It is estimated that the information desk receives 8,000 queries annually. A full-time staff member can handle about 20 queries per day. The employees at the facility typically use nine vacation days and take seven sick days during the year, and there are eleven holidays as well. How many full-time employees should the health care administrator include in the budget, taking into account the productivity adjustment? Round all figures to the nearest tenth and all percentages to the nearest point.

    a. 1.1
    b. 1.3
    c. 1.7
    d. 2.5

12. To what are the statistics referring that indicate one of every three men will develop benign prostate hypertrophy?

    a. Coincidence
    b. Prevalence
    c. Morbidity
    d. Incidence

13. Which data item is least likely to appear on the clinical forms of a patient in long-term care?

    a. Encounter record
    b. Registration record
    c. Medical history
    d. Progress notes

14. If a test produces 400 true positives, 350 true negatives, 50 false positives, and 20 false negatives, what is the sensitivity of the test? Round your answer to the nearest percentage point.

    a. 88%
    b. 90%
    c. 92%
    d. 95%

15. In which of the following situations would the burden of proof shift to the defendant in a malpractice suit?

    a. A patient under general anesthesia remains in a coma for several weeks.
    b. A patient finds that a surgical tool has been inadvertently sewn up into her body.
    c. A patient does not recover full range of motion after rotator-cuff surgery.
    d. Medication makes a patient nauseous.

16. Which government body is primarily responsible for standardizing health information?

   a. National Committee on Vital and Health Statistics
   b. American Health Information Management Association
   c. National Center for Health Statistics
   d. Health and Human Services Data Council

17. What is one advantage of bench research over clinical research?

   a. Bench research is less time-consuming.
   b. Bench research requires fewer participants.
   c. Bench research is less expensive.
   d. Bench research is less likely to be influenced by unpredictable behavior factors.

18. A hospital has average daily patient revenues of $32,000 and patient accounts receivable of $84,000. What is the hospital's ratio for days of revenue in patient accounts receivable? Round your answer to the nearest tenth.

   a. 0.4
   b. 2.6
   c. 8.4
   d. 3.2

19. For the month of July, the case mix value of a particular diagnosis-related group was 1.4, and 40 cases were recorded. What was the total value of service for July? Round your answer to the nearest whole number.

   a. 22
   b. 29
   c. 37
   d. 56

20. Which filing system would be most appropriate for a facility with a high risk of fire?

   a. Compressible filing system
   b. Open-shelf file system
   c. Filing cabinet
   d. Motorized revolving file system

21. What is the term for the percentage of people who have a disease at a particular time?

   a. Incidence rate
   b. Prevalence rate
   c. Morbidity rate
   d. Mortality rate

22. Which coding system is used most often by AIDS registries?

    a. SNOMED
    b. HCPCS
    c. DSM-5
    d. ICD-10-CM

23. During the month of March, a health care facility sees 140 total cases and provides services with a total value of 179. What is the case mix index for this period? Round your answer to the nearest tenth.

    a. 1.3
    b. 0.8
    c. 1.8
    d. 0.4

24. In health insurance, what is the name for an amendment that increases or decreases benefits?

    a. Deductible
    b. Rider
    c. Copayment
    d. Premium

25. Which of these scenarios illustrates ascertainment bias?

    a. Based on the answers given at the beginning of an interview, the interviewer tends to modify his or her style of questioning.
    b. A study is largely based on interviews, and the subjects tend to exaggerate the severity of their ailments.
    c. The subjects of a new research study have received a disproportionate amount of health treatment in the past.
    d. Two pathologists offer conflicting diagnoses when presented with the same set of specimens.

26. Which of the following pieces of data is only rarely on administrative forms for patients in hospice care?

    a. Transfer or referral form
    b. Consent to treatment
    c. Consent to special procedures
    d. Death certificate

27. Which type of data is a measure of blood pressure?

    a. Continuous data
    b. Discrete data
    c. Nominal data
    d. Ordinal data

28. During May, a 500-bed facility had 400 deaths, 2,000 other discharges, and 345 comorbidities. What was the comorbidity rate for this month, rounded to the nearest tenth of a percent?

    a. 20.8%
    b. 40.0%
    c. 17.3%
    d. 14.4%

29. If a test produces 200 true positives, 50 false negatives, 175 true negatives, and 40 false positives, what is the specificity of the test? Round your answer to the nearest percentage point.

    a. 27%
    b. 57%
    c. 81%
    d. 91%

30. In which cost allocation method does the indirect department that provides the most service to other departments and receives the least service from other indirect departments have its costs allocated first?

    a. Simultaneous-equations method
    b. Step-down method
    c. Double-distribution method
    d. All of the above

31. During the month of April, the pediatrics department of a hospital sees 25 patients, with an average length of stay of 3 days, and the internal medicine department sees 50 patients, with an average length of stay of 4 days. What is the weighted average length of stay for April? Round your answer to the nearest tenth.

    a. 0.5 days
    b. 3.7 days
    c. 4.4 days
    d. 5.4 days

32. In which numbering system does a patient retain the same number for each of his or her encounters?

    a. Serial-unit numbering
    b. Serial numbering
    c. Unit numbering
    d. All of the above

33. Which of the following is an advantage of the case-control study design?

    a. The case-control study design is less likely to be influenced by bias than the cohort study.

    b. It is easy to select an appropriate control group for a case-control study.

    c. It is easy to validate the information obtained from a case-control study.

    d. The case-control study design requires few subjects relative to other study designs.

34. In general examinations, dermatologists tend to overemphasize the significance of moles and ignore more subtle but equally worrisome phenomena. Which type of error does this scenario exemplify?

    a. Recency effect

    b. Central tendency error

    c. Halo effect

    d. Leniency bias

35. Which federal data set was established to enable comparison of outpatient care?

    a. Uniform Hospital Discharge Data Set (UHDDS)

    b. Uniform Ambulatory Core Data Set (UACDS)

    c. Minimum Data Set for Long-Term Care (MDS)

    d. Outcome and Assessment Information Set (OASIS)

36. Which word refers to a large outbreak of a contagious disease over a limited geographical region?

    a. Pandemic

    b. Epidemic

    c. Endemic

    d. Sporadic

37. The _____ of data is the degree to which it has appropriate specificity.

    a. granularity

    b. relevancy

    c. accuracy

    d. accessibility

38. In which site of care are patient records least likely to contain nursing notes?

    a. Behavioral health care

    b. Hospice care

    c. Acute care

    d. Ambulatory care

39. Which of the following are NOT a component of a PERT network?

a. Activities
b. Events
c. Goals
d. Reasons

40. Which form of planning has the briefest time horizon?

a. Tactical planning
b. Operational planning
c. Diagnostic planning
d. Strategic planning

41. Which of the following positions is most likely to be filled by several people in a large hospital?

a. Chief operating officer
b. Chief financial officer
c. Chief executive officer
d. Chief information officer

42. A 300-bed facility had 12,500 discharge days, 200 deaths, and 1,800 other discharges during the month of August. What was the average length of stay for August at this facility? Round your answer to the nearest hundredth.

a. 6.94
b. 4.79
c. 6.25
d. 62.50

43. Which MDS applies to acute care provision?

a. Minimum Data Set for Long-Term Care
b. Uniform Ambulatory Core Data Set
c. Outcome and Assessment Information Set
d. Uniform Hospital Discharge Data Set

44. Which of the following charts depicts the actual physical movements required for a process?

a. Flow process chart
b. Layout flowchart
c. Systems flowchart
d. Gantt chart

45. Which of the following is a disadvantage of prospective study?

a. Prospective study is expensive.
b. Prospective study only estimates relative risk.
c. Prospective study is subject to recall bias.
d. Prospective study is unable to determine whether the symptom preceded the disease.

46. Which piece of legislation established the National Practitioner Data Bank?

    a. Tax Equity and Fiscal Responsibility Act
    b. Health Care Quality Improvement Act
    c. Health Insurance Portability and Accountability Act
    d. Nursing Home Reform Act

47. Which micrographics option is best for very old records?

    a. CAR-roll microfilm
    b. CAR-jacket microfilm
    c. Roll microfilm
    d. Microfilm jackets

48. A health care facility has current assets of $500,000 and current liabilities of $200,000. What is the current ratio of the health care facility?

    a. 1.8
    b. 2.5
    c. 4.2
    d. 5.2

49. Which of the following is a keyed entry device?

    a. Mark-sense reader
    b. Optical scanner
    c. Bar code reader
    d. Light pen

50. A study focuses on determining the proportion of patients with dental problems whose care plans adhere to the American Dental Association's guidelines. Which dimension of performance is addressed by this study?

    a. Efficacy
    b. Appropriateness
    c. Continuity
    d. Efficiency

Answer Key and Explanations

1. A: The validity of this laboratory test is deficient. In laboratory research, *validity* is the extent to which a test measures what it is intended to measure. The *reliability* of the test is the extent to which it can be depended upon to give a consistent reading in different circumstances. The *specificity* of the test is the extent to which it correctly identifies all true noncases (that is, all true negatives and false positives). The sensitivity of the test is the extent to which it correctly identifies all true cases (that is, all true positives and false negatives).

2. D: Typically, the first step in a progressive disciplinary process is an oral warning. In most cases, a progressive discipline approach is most effective. It is important, however, that the sequence of gradually increasing punishments be made explicit to employees during orientation. The usual sequence of progressive discipline is oral warning, written reprimand, suspension, and finally, termination. A progressive discipline process gives the employee opportunities to rectify his or her behavior.

3. C: The patient's name must be collected during each visit to a health practitioner. Indeed, it is absolutely essential that this piece of data be recorded in the same way every time. For this reason, some organizations recommend using Social Security number rather than name because health care employees are less likely to make mistakes with a number then with the spelling of a name. The other answer choices represent pieces of data that should only be collected upon the first visit or when necessary. It is recommended that the patient's date of birth be recorded in the following order: four-digit year, two-digit month, and two-digit day. The precise categories for ethnicity are outlined by the Office of Management and Budget Directive 15. *Self-reported health status* is a general measure, often placed on a five-point scale (poor, fair, good, very good, and excellent).

4. C: The inpatient bed occupancy rate for January was about 89%. This census statistic is also called the *occupancy rate, occupancy percentage, or percentage of occupancy*. The inpatient bed occupancy rate is calculated by dividing the number of inpatient service days by the product of the number of beds and the number of days in the month and then multiplying by 100. So, for this question, inpatient bed occupancy rate is calculated $[11{,}000 \div (400 \times 31)] \times 100 = [11{,}000 \div 12{,}400] \times 100 = 0.887 \times 100 = 88.7\%$.

5. B: The most likely reason for the results in this scenario is nonresponse bias. *Nonresponse bias* occurs when it is probable that survey respondents will have significantly different characteristics than survey nonrespondents. In this scenario, it seems likely that cultural pressures would encourage people to underreport their alcohol consumption or for heavy drinkers to avoid reporting any consumption at all. *Diagnosis bias,* on the other hand, occurs when there is disagreement among professionals about the meaning of specimens collected during a research study. A *prevarication bias* exists when survey respondents embellish their answers, either by exaggerating their characteristics or providing obfuscating detail. *Survival bias*

111

occurs when the results of a study are influenced by the fact that the members of a population who are still alive are more likely to share certain characteristics. For instance, a study of 80-year-old lifelong smokers might produce a smaller-than-expected incidence of cancer for the simple reason that other lifelong smokers would have died of the disease by this age.

6. C: In this scenario, the administrator is using the quality improvement strategy of comparative benchmarking. In *comparative benchmarking,* an administrator compares a process in his or her business to a similar, but not exactly correspondent, process in another industry. Obviously, a hospital administrator will not use precisely the same strategy as a restaurant manager to increase customer flow, but the administrator may be able to obtain some insights from the comparison. The other two common types of benchmarking are performance and internal benchmarking. In *performance benchmarking,* also known as *competitive benchmarking,* administrators compare the performance of their organizations with the performance of leaders within their industry. In *performance benchmarking,* an organization looks at the exact same processes as performed by successful competitors. In *internal benchmarking,* administrators compare the performance of different departments within their own organizations. Obviously, this strategy is only effective when there are significant similarities in the processes performed by the departments.

7. D: *Quality assessment* is the form of management that makes the most use of statistical analysis. The other two common forms of management are utilization management and risk management. In *risk management,* the administrators are more likely to use occurrence screening, while in *utilization management,* they are more likely to use case management techniques. The purpose of quality assessment is to improve care and services by analyzing past performance. Utilization management focuses on effectively and efficiently using resources. Risk management is focused on avoiding liability.

8. B: The ICD-10-CM coding instrument is generally recommended for the principal diagnosis upon admittance to inpatient treatment. The International Classification of Diseases, 10th Edition, Clinical Modification (commonly known as the ICD-10-CM), is used to make the determination that will inform the patient's treatment from admission. The Systematized Nomenclature of Diseases and Operations (SNOMED) makes it possible for distant health care facilities to compare the treatment protocols and patient responses for common conditions. The Health Care Financing Administration Common Procedure Coding System (HCPCS) is used on the billing documents for inpatient, ambulatory, and surgical treatment. The Diagnostic and Statistical Manual of Mental Disorders (DSM-5) is the primary coding system for mental conditions.

9. A: The Health Insurance Portability and Accountability Act created a program for detecting fraudulent health plans. This act, passed in 1996 and implemented in 1998, generally improved the quality, access, and affordability of health insurance. The Nursing Home Reform Act, passed in 1987 and made effective in 1990, established minimum staffing requirements for long-term care facilities. The Patient Self-Determination Act, passed in 1990, mandated a wider dissemination of information to patients about their health options and rights. The Consolidated Omnibus Budget Reconciliation Act of 1985, commonly known as COBRA, established standards for the transfer and discharge of Medicaid and Medicare recipients.

10. D: A basic assumption of normative decision theory is that decision makers have total knowledge of the available options. Indeed, one of the main criticisms of normative decision theory is that it presumes an omniscience that no decision maker will have. *Normative decision theory* assumes that the decision maker will be able to maximize revenue because he or she will be able to survey available options with clear eyes and make the proper choice. *Behavioral decision theory,* on the other hand, acknowledges that decision makers will never have total knowledge of the situation and suggests that an emphasis should be placed on satisfying rather than optimal choices.

11. C: The health care administrator will need to include 1.7 full-time employees in the budget. This is a complex calculation, particularly when the productivity adjustment is made. To begin with, it is necessary to calculate the number of full-time employees that would be required if employees worked every day. This is done by first multiplying the number of queries an employee can handle by the number of days in a workweek and the number of weeks in a year: $20 \times 5 \times 52 = 5,200$. This is the total number of queries that a full-time employee could handle in a year if he or she worked every day. For this ideal scenario, the number of required employees can be calculated by dividing the total number of requests by the number of requests each employee can handle: $8,000 \div 5,200 = 1.5$. However, it is noted in the question that employees do not actually work every day. Full-time employees miss an average of 27 days each, which can be multiplied by the number of hours in a day to yield the total number of nonproductive hours: $27 \times 8 = 216$. The amount of actual productive time for each employee can then be calculated by subtracting these nonproductive hours from the ideal productive time, 2,080 (calculated by multiplying the number of hours in a workday by the number of days in a workweek by the number of weeks in a year): $2,080 - 216 = 1,864$. The productivity rate is calculated by dividing the amount of real productive time by the total possible amount of productive time: $1,864 \div 2080 = 0.896 = 90\%$. The actual number of full-time employees that need to be included in the budget can then be calculated by dividing the number of full-time employees required in the ideal productivity calculation by the productivity rate adjustment: $1.5/90\% = 1.7$ full-time employees.

12. B: Statistics that indicate one of every three men will develop benign prostate hypertrophy are referring to prevalence. *Prevalence* is the rate of the number of existing cases of a condition during a particular interval divided by the total population during that interval. In essence, it is the likelihood that a given member of a population would have a certain condition within a certain time. *Coincidence,* in health care, is the simultaneous occurrence of two distinct conditions. *Morbidity* is the extent to which a given population suffers from any illness, injury, or disability. The calculation of morbidity rate will typically include complication rates, comorbidity rates, and the incidence and prevalence rates of disease. Finally, in health care, *incidence* is the number of new cases of a particular condition during an interval; the incidence rate is calculated by dividing the number of new cases during the interval by the population during that interval.

13. A: Of the given data items, an encounter record is least likely to appear on the clinical forms of a patient in long-term care. Indeed, it is quite possible that this record will never appear on clinical forms for long-term care patients. The *encounter record* is a typical component of ambulatory care record keeping and is used during the billing process. It will include the basic diagnosis and treatment protocol. Registration records, medical history, and progress notes will almost always be a part of the clinical forms of a patient in long-term care. The *registration record* typically includes the basic diagnosis as well as the allergies and sensitivities of the patient. This record should be legible and should avoid symbols and abbreviations. The *medical history* is typically provided by the patient and should include the chief complaint, symptoms, history of illness, family history, and a basic review of systems. *Progress notes,* finally, keep a record of the patient's response to treatment.

14. D: If a test produces 400 true positives, 350 true negatives, 50 false positives, and 20 false negatives, the sensitivity of the test is 95%. The sensitivity of a test is calculated by dividing the number of true positives by the number of total positives (that is, the sum of true positives and false negatives). In this scenario, then, sensitivity is calculated 400/(400 +20) = 400/420 = 95.2%. The *sensitivity* of a test is the percentage of all true cases that the test identifies correctly.

15. B: If a patient discovers that a surgical tool has been inadvertently sewn up into her body, the burden of proof in the malpractice suit shifts to the defendant. This shift is based on the legal concept of *res ipsa loquitur,* or "a situation that speaks for itself." In this case, it is obvious that the nature of the injury indicates negligence and that the plaintiff could have had no role in her injury. In order for the burden of proof to shift to the defendant in a malpractice suit, it must be clear that the injury would not have occurred without negligence that the defendant was totally in control of the process that caused the injury, and that the plaintiff made no contribution to the injury. Of the answer choices, only B meets all of these criteria.

16. A: The National Committee on Vital and Health Statistics (NCVHS) is primarily responsible for standardizing health information. The NCVHS is a component of the department of Health and Human Services. It encourages public and private entities to collaborate on a uniform and efficient health information system. The American Health Information Management Association (AHIMA) is a professional development organization that offers training, certification, and research opportunities to those who are interested. The National Center for Health Statistics (NCHS) is a division of the Centers for Disease Control and Prevention (CDC). The NCHS is an aggregator and disseminator of vital and health statistics. The Health and

Human Services Data Council organizes the data collection efforts in both medical and nonmedical areas.

17. D: One advantage of bench research over clinical research is that it is less likely to be influenced by unpredictable behavior factors. *Bench research* takes place in a laboratory, while *clinical research* is performed with patients who have already manifested the condition being studied. In some cases, bench research may be less time-consuming, require fewer participants, or be less expensive, but this is not always the case. However, because bench research is conducted under controlled conditions, it is much less likely to be influenced by unpredictable or unexpected behavior factors.

18. B: The hospital's ratio for days of revenue in patient accounts receivable is 2.6. This ratio is calculated by dividing accounts receivable by the average daily revenue. In this scenario, then, the calculation is 84,000/32,000 = 2.6. The ratio for days of revenue in patient accounts receivable indicates how long it takes the hospital to collect payment or the time over which the hospital is willing to extend credit.

19. D: The total value of service for July was 56. Total value of service is calculated by multiplying case mix value by the number of cases recorded during the period. So, in this scenario, the calculation would be 1.4 × 40 = 56.

20. C: A filing cabinet system would be most appropriate for a facility with a high risk of fire. Filing cabinets are widely available in fireproof versions and generally are able to protect important records from environmental degradation. However, these cabinets can take up a great deal of space and, typically, can only be opened one drawer at a time. A *compressible filing system,* on the other hand, is a manual or motorized system of parallel open-shelf files that move back and forth to create an opening. Compressible filing systems save a great deal of space but can generate high maintenance costs. An *open-shelf filing system* is similar to a set of bookshelves: There is easy access to every file within the system, but all the records are open to environmental damage. A *motorized revolving file system,* finally, resembles a Ferris wheel. The systems are very space efficient, but they are also precarious and must be kept organized in order to function properly.

21. B: *Prevalence rate* is the percentage of people who have a disease at a particular time. The *incidence rate* is calculated as the number of new cases of a disease during a specific interval divided by the total population during that interval. The *morbidity rate* is essentially the rate of complications for patients, though it should be noted that this rate also includes the prevalence and incidence of disease as well as the comorbidity rate. The *mortality rate* could be any of a set of death rates, including the infant death rate, net death rate, or gross death rate.

22. D: The ICD-10-CM coding system is used most often by AIDS registries. It is extremely important for health officials to monitor the spread and pattern of AIDS incidences. The International Classification of Diseases, 10th Edition, Clinical Modification (ICD-10-CM), is the preferred coding system for admission. The

Systematized Nomenclature of Diseases and Operations (SNOMED) enables comparison of the treatment protocols for common ailments at disparate facilities. The Health Care Financing Administration Common Procedure Coding System (HCPCS) is commonly used by the billing departments of health care facilities. The Diagnostic and Statistical Manual of Mental Disorders (DSM-5) is the primary coding system and repository of diagnostic criteria for mental conditions.

23. A: The case mix index for this period is 1.3. The case mix index is calculated by dividing the total value of service by the total number of cases. In this case, then, the calculation is 179 ÷ 140 = 1.3. Determining the case mix index enables the health care facility to identify how well resources are being used in the treatment of particular ailments.

24. B: In health insurance, a *rider* is an amendment that increases or decreases benefits. A *deductible* is the minimum amount that the beneficiary of an insurance policy must incur before the insurance provider will pay for the remaining treatment. A *copayment* is a system in which the subscriber pays a certain amount out of his or her own pocket for every encounter with the health care system, with the remaining payment provided by the insurance company. A *premium*, finally, is a fixed payment made regularly to maintain insurance coverage.

25. C: A scenario in which the subjects of a new research study receive a disproportionate amount of health treatment is an illustration of ascertainment bias. *Ascertainment bias* is the tendency of researchers to more often select research subjects who receive a greater amount of medical treatment. This often occurs when the volunteer population of a research study is likely to be composed of people with special interests in physical fitness or nutrition. When the interviewer modifies his or her style of questioning based on the answers given early in the interview, this is an example of *interviewer bias*. Interviewer bias can be resolved by standardizing the question sequence. When subjects are apt to exaggerate the severity of their ailments, this is an illustration of *prevarication bias*. Prevarication bias is especially common in situations where research subjects have some incentive to manifest a particular medical condition, as for instance when they are receiving disability compensation. When two pathologists offer conflicting diagnoses of the same specimens, this is an example of *diagnosis bias*. Diagnosis bias can often be resolved by preventing the pathologists from knowing the provenance of the specimens.

26. C: The consent to special procedures is only rarely included on administrative forms for patients in hospice care. This is for obvious reasons, as patients who have entered hospice care have decided to eschew unlimited life-prolonging interventions in favor of a more comfortable death. It is not uncommon, however, for hospice patients to complete consents to treatment as it is important for legal reasons for them to be explicit about the steps that should be taken in emergency situations. Because a patient in hospice care is typically close to death, it is not abnormal for a template version of the death certificate to be kept in the patient's records. Finally, a hospice patient may have a transfer or referral form in his or her records in case the patient needs to receive palliative care elsewhere.

27. A: Blood pressure measurements are an example of continuous data. *Continuous data* has the potential to carry on infinitely in a meaningful sense. Weight and cost are two classic examples of continuous data as, theoretically, there is no upper limit to either. *Discrete data,* on the other hand, consists of meaningful whole numbers with a possibly unknown but extant upper limit. An example of discrete data would be the number of patients admitted by a health care facility during a particular interval. *Nominal data* is simply the set of numbers assigned to different categories. In nominal data sets, the exact values assigned are arbitrary. For instance, there is no real reason why females would be coded as 0 and males coded as 1, and not vice versa. *Ordinal data,* finally, indicates the position or rank of the data within a value set. A common example of ordinal data is the five-point self-assessment scale, on which patients describe their current health status.

28. D: The comorbidity rate for this facility during May was 14.4%. *Comorbidity rate* is a condition that the patient has upon being admitted, that is different from the condition for which the patient is being admitted, and that increases the patient's stay by at least a day three-quarters of the time. Comorbidity rate is calculated by dividing the total number of comorbidities by the total number of discharges, including deaths, and then multiplying the quotient by 100. So, in this scenario, comorbidity rate would be calculated $[345 \div (400 + 2000)] \times 100 = [345 \div 2400] \times 100 = 0.14375 \times 100 = 14.375\%$, or 14.4%.

29. C: If a test produces 200 true positives, 50 false negatives, 175 true negatives, and 40 false positives, the specificity of the test is 81%. The *specificity* of a test is the percentage of all true noncases that are identified. In other words, specificity is the success of the test at identifying those members of the population that do not have the condition. Specificity is calculated by dividing the number of true negatives by the total number of noncases (that is, the sum of true negatives and false positives). In this scenario, specificity is calculated $175/(175 + 40) = 175/215 = 81\%$.

30. B: In the *step-down method* of cost allocation, the indirect department that provides the most service to other departments and receives the least service from other indirect departments has its costs allocated first. The step-down method is the cost allocation method used by Medicare in its requirements for cost reporting. For this and other reasons, it is the most common method of cost allocation. The *simultaneous-equations method* requires the use of complex software programs and may require up to twelve different cost distributions. In the *double-distribution method,* a nonlinear allocation of costs is assumed, and it is acknowledged that some indirect departments must be allocated to smaller departments before their costs are fully allocated.

31. B: The weighted average length of stay for April is 3.7 days. *Weighted average length of stay* is a good measure for assessing the average length of stay per patient. It is a more detailed metric than a simple average of the lengths of stay in each department. Weighted average length of stay is calculated by adding up the products of the number of patients and the average length of stay within each department and then dividing this sum by the total number of patients. So, in this case, weighted average length of stay would be calculated (25 × 3 + 50 × 4) ÷ (25 + 50) = (75 + 200) ÷ 75 = 3.7.

32. C: In *a unit numbering system,* the patient contains the same number for each of his or her encounters. Each patient's record will be filed according to his or her unit number. In both the *serial and serial-unit numbering systems,* a patient will receive a new number for each encounter. Many health care facilities find that adopting a unit numbering system eliminates a great deal of work and prevents file folders from being spread out over disparate locations.

33. D: One advantage of the case-control design is that it requires few subjects relative to other study designs. Some other advantages of this study design are that it is relatively inexpensive, allows the use of already existing records, and poses only a slight risk to subjects. Case-control studies also produce results faster than prospective or cohort studies. However, case-control studies may easily be influenced by recall bias, and it can be very difficult to select an appropriate control group for such a study. Also, validating the information acquired during a case-control study may be difficult.

34. C: The tendency of dermatologists to overemphasize moles during general examinations is an example of the halo effect. The *halo effect* is the tendency to allow perception to become dominated by a single characteristic of the research subject. Metastudies of medical research have indicated that the halo effect is the most difficult bias to eradicate. *Central tendency error* is a tendency to group subjects in the middle of the evaluation range. The central tendency error is especially common in situations where the evaluator is subject to social pressures, as for instance, in situations where he or she is evaluating peers and does not wish to favor some subjects over others. The *recency effect* is a tendency to place undue influence on the most recent events. Recency effect is most problematic when the evaluator surveys a number of samples before rendering a judgment on all of them. Finally, the *leniency bias,* conversely known as the *strictness bias,* is an evaluator's individual tendency to be too permissive or harsh in his or her judgments.

35. B: The Uniform Ambulatory Core Data Set (UACDS) was devised to enable comparison of data from various patients in outpatient care. The Uniform Hospital Discharge Data Set (UHDDS) is the common set of data collected for inpatients. It is used by both federal and state agencies. The Minimum Data Set for Long-Term Care (MDS) is a wide-ranging functional assessment for patients in long-term care. The Outcome and Assessment Information Set (OASIS) is the primary basis for assessing patient outcomes. It is also a general assessment for adult patients in home care.

36. B: An *epidemic* is a large outbreak of a contagious disease over a geographical region. A *pandemic,* meanwhile, is a massive outbreak of a contagious disease over a large geographic area. *Endemic* means prevalent in or restricted to a particular region or population. This adjective is often used to describe medical conditions. *Sporadic* is also used frequently in this context: It means occurring or appearing in irregular intervals.

37. A: The *granularity* of data is the degree to which it has appropriate specificity. The *relevancy* of data is the extent to which it applies to the process or function for which it was collected. The *accuracy* of data is its correctness. The *accessibility* of data is the ease and legality with which it may be collected.

38. D: Patient records related to ambulatory care are the least likely to contain nursing notes. Nursing notes outline the patient's condition and treatment protocol in specific terms. A set of nursing notes typically includes an admission note and a summary of all nursing interventions, including a description of the patient's response. The concluding document in a series of nursing notes will be the discharge record. Because nursing notes pertain explicitly to inpatient treatment, they will rarely be created for ambulatory patients.

39. D: Reasons are not a component of a PERT network. The acronym PERT stands for Program Evaluation Review Technique. This methodology was developed to help administrators sequence complex processes. The three components of a PERT network are goals, events, and activities. The *goal* is the basic intention of the network. The *events* in the network are specific activities or groups of activities that will contribute to the achievement of the goal. *Activities* are the tasks that must be performed in order to move from one event to the other.

40. B: Of all forms of planning, operational planning has the briefest time horizon. It is typical for an operational plan to extend only over a few weeks or months. The completion of an *operational plan* is a step toward the completion of a tactical plan, which extends over a slightly longer time horizon. *Tactical plans* typically include several operational plans. Similarly, *strategic plans* typically include several tactical plans. A strategic plan has the longest time horizon, extending over multiple years in many cases.

41. A: Of the given positions, chief operating officer is most likely to be filled by several people in a large hospital. The chief operating officer or officers will report directly to the chief executive officer. *Chief operating officers* are responsible for managing the performance of individual departments and ensuring that employees always act in consonance with the organizational goals. The *chief financial officer,* also known as the *director of finance,* is responsible for managing the fiscal activities of the institution. The *chief executive officer* is appointed by the board of directors and is the principal authority for the institution. The *chief information officer* is responsible for managing the organization's information resources. This individual's purview includes the financial, clinical, and administrative information operations.

42. C: The average length of stay is calculated by dividing the number of discharge days by the number of discharges, including deaths. In this scenario, then, average length of stay would be $12,500 \div (200 + 1,800) = 12,500 \div 2,000 = 6.25$. In other words, during the month of August, patients stayed at this health care facility an average of 6 ¼ days.

43. D: The Uniform Hospital Discharge Data Set (UHDDS) is the appropriate minimum data set (MDS) for acute care provision. This data set is used by both federal and state agencies to standardize information for inpatients. It is maintained by the National Committee on Vital Health Statistics. The Minimum Data Set for Long-Term Care (MDS) is a more wide-ranging functional assessment for long-term care patients. The Uniform Ambulatory Core Data Set (UACDS) provides health care facilities the chance to compare data for ambulatory patients. The Outcome and Assessment Information Set (OASIS) is the MDS for home health care and the primary source of information on long-term patient outcomes.

44. B: A *layout flowchart* depicts the actual physical movements required for a process. These charts, which are also known as *movement diagrams,* are used to demonstrate the path of a particular document or employee during the course of a typical process. The layout flowchart is often able to identify redundancies or bottlenecks. A *flow process chart,* on the other hand, is a basic summation of the steps involved in a particular work process. A *systems flowchart* depicts the path of information through a system. A *Gantt chart,* finally, organizes the schedule of a complex process.

45. A: One disadvantage of prospective study is that it is very expensive. Some other disadvantages of this type of system are that it takes a long time to produce results, and it may easily be influenced by unpredictable changes in the environment or the behavior patterns of participants. Also, prospective study is not good at obtaining information about rare diseases. However, prospective study is able to determine relative risk exactly, and it is notably devoid of recall bias. Moreover, a prospective study is usually able to identify whether the symptom preceded the disease.

46. B: The Health Care Quality Improvement Act established the National Practitioner Data Bank in 1986. The National Practitioner Data Bank assembles and disseminates information about incompetent or malpracticing health care service providers. The Health Insurance Portability and Accountability Act improved the quality of health insurance and created a program for detecting fraud and abuse in health plans. The Tax Equity and Fiscal Responsibility Act (TEFRA) made significant changes to the Medicare reimbursement structure. The Nursing Home Reform Act established minimum staffing requirements for long-term care facilities.

47. C: Roll microfilm is the best micrographics option for very old records. A *roll microfilm* functions in much the same way as a traditional filmstrip: Documents are represented sequentially and are numbered. A roll microfilm system can hold about 2,400 images. In a *computer-assisted retrieval (CAR)-roll microfilm system,* images are represented in a similar way, but the microfilm can be updated. In a *computer-assisted retrieval (CAR)-jacket microfilm system,* 4 x 6 film holders can contain 70 individual images; each set of prenumbered film is contained in a specific channel. In a *microfilm jacket system,* each holder contains all the records for a single patient. This is the most appropriate system for health care facilities in which individual patients receive frequent treatment.

48. B: The current ratio of the health care facility is 2.5. *Current ratio,* which is one of the most common liquidity ratios used in finance, is simply a comparison of current assets with current liabilities. In this case, then, it is calculated 500,000/200,000 = 2.5. Values for current assets and current liabilities are obtainable from the balance sheet. The general point of the current ratio is to indicate whether the business has enough cash or liquid assets to cover its short-term obligations.

49. D: A light pen is a keyed entry device. A *keyed entry device* uses a graphical user interface, similar to a Windows desktop. A light pen is a special instrument that is applied directly to the display screen to enter information. Mark-sense readers, optical scanners, and bar code readers are all examples of scanned entry devices. A *scanned entry device* uses a piece of sensory equipment to read the information into its memory system. In a *mark-sense reader system,* employees use a pencil to darken circles on a form, which is then fed into a machine and entered into memory. A mark-sense reader functions much like a standardized multiple-choice test. An *optical scanner* transmits the image of a paper document into computer memory. A *bar code reader* obtains information from a series of varying black vertical stripes on the document. Bar codes are considered to be extremely accurate, though they may be time-consuming to create.

50. A: The dimension of performance addressed by this study is efficacy. In the provision of health services, *efficacy* is the extent to which an activity achieves its intended outcome. The study in this question then, is measuring the efficacy of the guidelines provided by the American Dental Association. It is important for a medical service authority to understand how often and how exactly its recommendations are followed. The *appropriateness* of an activity is the extent to which it applies to the clinical needs of the patient. The *continuity* of the study is the extent to which multiple health care providers are able to coordinate and maintain consistent therapy for patients over a long duration. Finally, the *efficiency* of health care activity is the extent to which the desired outcomes are achieved with a minimum use of resources.

How to Overcome Test Anxiety

Just the thought of taking a test is enough to make most people a little nervous. A test is an important event that can have a long-term impact on your future, so it's important to take it seriously and it's natural to feel anxious about performing well. But just because anxiety is normal, that doesn't mean that it's helpful in test taking, or that you should simply accept it as part of your life. Anxiety can have a variety of effects. These effects can be mild, like making you feel slightly nervous, or severe, like blocking your ability to focus or remember even a simple detail.

If you experience test anxiety—whether severe or mild—it's important to know how to beat it. To discover this, first you need to understand what causes test anxiety.

Causes of Test Anxiety

While we often think of anxiety as an uncontrollable emotional state, it can actually be caused by simple, practical things. One of the most common causes of test anxiety is that a person does not feel adequately prepared for their test. This feeling can be the result of many different issues such as poor study habits or lack of organization, but the most common culprit is time management. Starting to study too late, failing to organize your study time to cover all of the material, or being distracted while you study will mean that you're not well prepared for the test. This may lead to cramming the night before, which will cause you to be physically and mentally exhausted for the test. Poor time management also contributes to feelings of stress, fear, and hopelessness as you realize you are not well prepared but don't know what to do about it.

Other times, test anxiety is not related to your preparation for the test but comes from unresolved fear. This may be a past failure on a test, or poor performance on tests in general. It may come from comparing yourself to others who seem to be performing better or from the stress of living up to expectations. Anxiety may be driven by fears of the future—how failure on this test would affect your educational and career goals. These fears are often completely irrational, but they can still negatively impact your test performance.

> **Review Video: 3 Reasons You Have Test Anxiety**
> Visit mometrix.com/academy and enter code: 428468

Elements of Test Anxiety

As mentioned earlier, test anxiety is considered to be an emotional state, but it has physical and mental components as well. Sometimes you may not even realize that you are suffering from test anxiety until you notice the physical symptoms. These can include trembling hands, rapid heartbeat, sweating, nausea, and tense muscles. Extreme anxiety may lead to fainting or vomiting. Obviously, any of these symptoms can have a negative impact on testing. It is important to recognize them as soon as they begin to occur so that you can address the problem before it damages your performance.

Review Video: 3 Ways to Tell You Have Test Anxiety
Visit mometrix.com/academy and enter code: 927847

The mental components of test anxiety include trouble focusing and inability to remember learned information. During a test, your mind is on high alert, which can help you recall information and stay focused for an extended period of time. However, anxiety interferes with your mind's natural processes, causing you to blank out, even on the questions you know well. The strain of testing during anxiety makes it difficult to stay focused, especially on a test that may take several hours. Extreme anxiety can take a huge mental toll, making it difficult not only to recall test information but even to understand the test questions or pull your thoughts together.

Review Video: How Test Anxiety Affects Memory
Visit mometrix.com/academy and enter code: 609003

Effects of Test Anxiety

Test anxiety is like a disease—if left untreated, it will get progressively worse. Anxiety leads to poor performance, and this reinforces the feelings of fear and failure, which in turn lead to poor performances on subsequent tests. It can grow from a mild nervousness to a crippling condition. If allowed to progress, test anxiety can have a big impact on your schooling, and consequently on your future.

Test anxiety can spread to other parts of your life. Anxiety on tests can become anxiety in any stressful situation, and blanking on a test can turn into panicking in a job situation. But fortunately, you don't have to let anxiety rule your testing and determine your grades. There are a number of relatively simple steps you can take to move past anxiety and function normally on a test and in the rest of life.

Review Video: How Test Anxiety Impacts Your Grades
Visit mometrix.com/academy and enter code: 939819

Physical Steps for Beating Test Anxiety

While test anxiety is a serious problem, the good news is that it can be overcome. It doesn't have to control your ability to think and remember information. While it may take time, you can begin taking steps today to beat anxiety.

Just as your first hint that you may be struggling with anxiety comes from the physical symptoms, the first step to treating it is also physical. Rest is crucial for having a clear, strong mind. If you are tired, it is much easier to give in to anxiety. But if you establish good sleep habits, your body and mind will be ready to perform optimally, without the strain of exhaustion. Additionally, sleeping well helps you to retain information better, so you're more likely to recall the answers when you see the test questions.

Getting good sleep means more than going to bed on time. It's important to allow your brain time to relax. Take study breaks from time to time so it doesn't get overworked, and don't study right before bed. Take time to rest your mind before trying to rest your body, or you may find it difficult to fall asleep.

Review Video: <u>The Importance of Sleep for Your Brain</u>
Visit mometrix.com/academy and enter code: 319338

Along with sleep, other aspects of physical health are important in preparing for a test. Good nutrition is vital for good brain function. Sugary foods and drinks may give a burst of energy but this burst is followed by a crash, both physically and emotionally. Instead, fuel your body with protein and vitamin-rich foods.

Also, drink plenty of water. Dehydration can lead to headaches and exhaustion, especially if your brain is already under stress from the rigors of the test. Particularly if your test is a long one, drink water during the breaks. And if possible, take an energy-boosting snack to eat between sections.

Review Video: <u>How Diet Can Affect your Mood</u>
Visit mometrix.com/academy and enter code: 624317

Along with sleep and diet, a third important part of physical health is exercise. Maintaining a steady workout schedule is helpful, but even taking 5-minute study breaks to walk can help get your blood pumping faster and clear your head. Exercise also releases endorphins, which contribute to a positive feeling and can help combat test anxiety.

When you nurture your physical health, you are also contributing to your mental health. If your body is healthy, your mind is much more likely to be healthy as well. So take time to rest, nourish your body with healthy food and water, and get moving as much as possible. Taking these physical steps will make you stronger and more able to take the mental steps necessary to overcome test anxiety.

Mental Steps for Beating Test Anxiety

Working on the mental side of test anxiety can be more challenging, but as with the physical side, there are clear steps you can take to overcome it. As mentioned earlier, test anxiety often stems from lack of preparation, so the obvious solution is to prepare for the test. Effective studying may be the most important weapon you have for beating test anxiety, but you can and should employ several other mental tools to combat fear.

First, boost your confidence by reminding yourself of past success—tests or projects that you aced. If you're putting as much effort into preparing for this test as you did for those, there's no reason you should expect to fail here. Work hard to prepare; then trust your preparation.

Second, surround yourself with encouraging people. It can be helpful to find a study group, but be sure that the people you're around will encourage a positive attitude. If you spend time with others who are anxious or cynical, this will only contribute to your own anxiety. Look for others who are motivated to study hard from a desire to succeed, not from a fear of failure.

Third, reward yourself. A test is physically and mentally tiring, even without anxiety, and it can be helpful to have something to look forward to. Plan an activity following the test, regardless of the outcome, such as going to a movie or getting ice cream.

When you are taking the test, if you find yourself beginning to feel anxious, remind yourself that you know the material. Visualize successfully completing the test. Then take a few deep, relaxing breaths and return to it. Work through the questions carefully but with confidence, knowing that you are capable of succeeding.

Developing a healthy mental approach to test taking will also aid in other areas of life. Test anxiety affects more than just the actual test—it can be damaging to your mental health and even contribute to depression. It's important to beat test anxiety before it becomes a problem for more than testing.

Study Strategy

Being prepared for the test is necessary to combat anxiety, but what does being prepared look like? You may study for hours on end and still not feel prepared. What you need is a strategy for test prep. The next few pages outline our recommended steps to help you plan out and conquer the challenge of preparation.

STEP 1: SCOPE OUT THE TEST

Learn everything you can about the format (multiple choice, essay, etc.) and what will be on the test. Gather any study materials, course outlines, or sample exams that may be available. Not only will this help you to prepare, but knowing what to expect can help to alleviate test anxiety.

STEP 2: MAP OUT THE MATERIAL

Look through the textbook or study guide and make note of how many chapters or sections it has. Then divide these over the time you have. For example, if a book has 15 chapters and you have five days to study, you need to cover three chapters each day. Even better, if you have the time, leave an extra day at the end for overall review after you have gone through the material in depth.

If time is limited, you may need to prioritize the material. Look through it and make note of which sections you think you already have a good grasp on, and which need review. While you are studying, skim quickly through the familiar sections and take more time on the challenging parts. Write out your plan so you don't get lost as you go. Having a written plan also helps you feel more in control of the study, so anxiety is less likely to arise from feeling overwhelmed at the amount to cover.

STEP 3: GATHER YOUR TOOLS

Decide what study method works best for you. Do you prefer to highlight in the book as you study and then go back over the highlighted portions? Or do you type out notes of the important information? Or is it helpful to make flashcards that you can carry with you? Assemble the pens, index cards, highlighters, post-it notes, and any other materials you may need so you won't be distracted by getting up to find things while you study.

If you're having a hard time retaining the information or organizing your notes, experiment with different methods. For example, try color-coding by subject with colored pens, highlighters, or post-it notes. If you learn better by hearing, try recording yourself reading your notes so you can listen while in the car, working out, or simply sitting at your desk. Ask a friend to quiz you from your flashcards, or try teaching someone the material to solidify it in your mind.

STEP 4: CREATE YOUR ENVIRONMENT

It's important to avoid distractions while you study. This includes both the obvious distractions like visitors and the subtle distractions like an uncomfortable chair (or a too-comfortable couch that makes you want to fall asleep). Set up the best study environment possible: good lighting and a comfortable work area. If background music helps you focus, you may want to turn it on, but otherwise keep the room quiet. If you are using a computer to take notes, be sure you don't have any other windows open, especially applications like social media, games, or anything else that could distract you. Silence your phone and turn off notifications. Be sure to keep water close by so you stay hydrated while you study (but avoid unhealthy drinks and snacks).

Also, take into account the best time of day to study. Are you freshest first thing in the morning? Try to set aside some time then to work through the material. Is your mind clearer in the afternoon or evening? Schedule your study session then. Another method is to study at the same time of day that you will take the test, so that your brain gets used to working on the material at that time and will be ready to focus at test time.

STEP 5: STUDY!

Once you have done all the study preparation, it's time to settle into the actual studying. Sit down, take a few moments to settle your mind so you can focus, and begin to follow your study plan. Don't give in to distractions or let yourself procrastinate. This is your time to prepare so you'll be ready to fearlessly approach the test. Make the most of the time and stay focused.

Of course, you don't want to burn out. If you study too long you may find that you're not retaining the information very well. Take regular study breaks. For example, taking five minutes out of every hour to walk briskly, breathing deeply and swinging your arms, can help your mind stay fresh.

As you get to the end of each chapter or section, it's a good idea to do a quick review. Remind yourself of what you learned and work on any difficult parts. When you feel that you've mastered the material, move on to the next part. At the end of your study session, briefly skim through your notes again.

But while review is helpful, cramming last minute is NOT. If at all possible, work ahead so that you won't need to fit all your study into the last day. Cramming overloads your brain with more information than it can process and retain, and your tired mind may struggle to recall even previously learned information when it is overwhelmed with last-minute study. Also, the urgent nature of cramming and the stress placed on your brain contribute to anxiety. You'll be more likely to go to the test feeling unprepared and having trouble thinking clearly.

So don't cram, and don't stay up late before the test, even just to review your notes at a leisurely pace. Your brain needs rest more than it needs to go over the information again. In fact, plan to finish your studies by noon or early afternoon the day before the test. Give your brain the rest of the day to relax or focus on other things, and get a good night's sleep. Then you will be fresh for the test and better able to recall what you've studied.

STEP 6: TAKE A PRACTICE TEST

Many courses offer sample tests, either online or in the study materials. This is an excellent resource to check whether you have mastered the material, as well as to prepare for the test format and environment.

Check the test format ahead of time: the number of questions, the type (multiple choice, free response, etc.), and the time limit. Then create a plan for working through them. For example, if you have 30 minutes to take a 60-question test, your limit is 30 seconds per question. Spend less time on the questions you know well so that you can take more time on the difficult ones.

If you have time to take several practice tests, take the first one open book, with no time limit. Work through the questions at your own pace and make sure you fully understand them. Gradually work up to taking a test under test conditions: sit at a desk with all study materials put away and set a timer. Pace yourself to make sure you finish the test with time to spare and go back to check your answers if you have time.

After each test, check your answers. On the questions you missed, be sure you understand why you missed them. Did you misread the question (tests can use tricky wording)? Did you forget the information? Or was it something you hadn't learned? Go back and study any shaky areas that the practice tests reveal.

Taking these tests not only helps with your grade, but also aids in combating test anxiety. If you're already used to the test conditions, you're less likely to worry about it, and working through tests until you're scoring well gives you a confidence boost. Go through the practice tests until you feel comfortable, and then you can go into the test knowing that you're ready for it.

Test Tips

On test day, you should be confident, knowing that you've prepared well and are ready to answer the questions. But aside from preparation, there are several test day strategies you can employ to maximize your performance.

First, as stated before, get a good night's sleep the night before the test (and for several nights before that, if possible). Go into the test with a fresh, alert mind rather than staying up late to study.

Try not to change too much about your normal routine on the day of the test. It's important to eat a nutritious breakfast, but if you normally don't eat breakfast at all, consider eating just a protein bar. If you're a coffee drinker, go ahead and have your normal coffee. Just make sure you time it so that the caffeine doesn't wear off right in the middle of your test. Avoid sugary beverages, and drink enough water to stay hydrated but not so much that you need a restroom break 10 minutes into the test. If your test isn't first thing in the morning, consider going for a walk or doing a light workout before the test to get your blood flowing.

Allow yourself enough time to get ready, and leave for the test with plenty of time to spare so you won't have the anxiety of scrambling to arrive in time. Another reason to be early is to select a good seat. It's helpful to sit away from doors and windows, which can be distracting. Find a good seat, get out your supplies, and settle your mind before the test begins.

When the test begins, start by going over the instructions carefully, even if you already know what to expect. Make sure you avoid any careless mistakes by following the directions.

Then begin working through the questions, pacing yourself as you've practiced. If you're not sure on an answer, don't spend too much time on it, and don't let it shake your confidence. Either skip it and come back later, or eliminate as many wrong answers as possible and guess among the remaining ones. Don't dwell on these questions as you continue—put them out of your mind and focus on what lies ahead.

Be sure to read all of the answer choices, even if you're sure the first one is the right answer. Sometimes you'll find a better one if you keep reading. But don't second-guess yourself if you do immediately know the answer. Your gut instinct is usually right. Don't let test anxiety rob you of the information you know.

If you have time at the end of the test (and if the test format allows), go back and review your answers. Be cautious about changing any, since your first instinct tends to be correct, but make sure you didn't misread any of the questions or accidentally mark the wrong answer choice. Look over any you skipped and make an educated guess.

At the end, leave the test feeling confident. You've done your best, so don't waste time worrying about your performance or wishing you could change anything. Instead, celebrate the successful completion of this test. And finally, use this test to learn how to deal with anxiety even better next time.

> **Review Video: 5 Tips to Beat Test Anxiety**
> Visit mometrix.com/academy and enter code: 570656

Important Qualification

Not all anxiety is created equal. If your test anxiety is causing major issues in your life beyond the classroom or testing center, or if you are experiencing troubling physical symptoms related to your anxiety, it may be a sign of a serious physiological or psychological condition. If this sounds like your situation, we strongly encourage you to seek professional help.

Thank You

We at Mometrix would like to extend our heartfelt thanks to you, our friend and patron, for allowing us to play a part in your journey. It is a privilege to serve people from all walks of life who are unified in their commitment to building the best future they can for themselves.

The preparation you devote to these important testing milestones may be the most valuable educational opportunity you have for making a real difference in your life. We encourage you to put your heart into it—that feeling of succeeding, overcoming, and yes, conquering will be well worth the hours you've invested.

We want to hear your story, your struggles and your successes, and if you see any opportunities for us to improve our materials so we can help others even more effectively in the future, please share that with us as well. **The team at Mometrix would be absolutely thrilled to hear from you!** So please, send us an email (support@mometrix.com) and let's stay in touch.

> **If you'd like some additional help, check out these other resources we offer for your exam:**
> http://MometrixFlashcards.com/AHIMA

Additional Bonus Material

Due to our efforts to try to keep this book to a manageable length, we've created a link that will give you access to all of your additional bonus material.

Please visit http://www.mometrix.com/bonus948/rhit to access the information.